THE CARE OF CHILDREN

Elizabeth Robinson Scovil

Superintendent of the Newport Hospital, and
One of the Associate Editors of the Ladies' Home Journal

Edited By
Jonathan D. Savage, Esq.
Mikesch Muecke, Ph.D..
Judy Berthiaume, LPN

Originally published in 1894

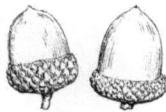

HOG PRESS

Hog Press
an imprint of Culicidae Press
PO Box 5069
Madison, WI 53705-5069
USA
culicidaepress.com
editor@culicidaepress.com

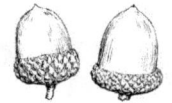

HOG PRESS

THE CARE OF CHILDREN
Copyright © 2024 by Elizabeth Robinson Scovil

ISBN: 978-1-941892-87-9

Our books may be purchased in bulk for promotional, educational or business use. Please contact your local bookseller or the Culicidae Press Sales Department at +1-515-462-0278 or by email at sales@culicidaepress.com

x.com/culicidaepress – facebook.com/culicidaepress
threads.net/culicidaepress – instagram.com/culicidaepress

Designed by polytekton ©2024
Cover design by Sarah Burkey

Dedication

I dedicate my efforts on this book to my dear friends Karen and Carl. Although neither has, to date, read this book, they clearly made the sacrifices and shared the universal wisdom detailed here in raising and caring for their six children, two adopted from overseas. The children (now adults) are solid citizens of our nation and our world, are of the faith of and follow the values taught by this book's author, and remain deeply grateful to their parents and family legacy. Awesome to see.

As a matter of record, Karen is a fifth cousin, three times removed, of the author Elizabeth Robinson Scovil. We discovered this just prior to going to press. High-quality lineage runs deep among these relatives.

Jonathan Savage

Disclaimer

This book is an edited reprint of the original titled *The Care of Children*, authored by Elizabeth Robinson Scovil. The book was initially printed and copyrighted in 1894, well over one hundred years ago.

Ms. Scovil's writings contain practical advice and proven wisdom for readers of the late nineteenth and early twentieth century. The book cannot and should not in any way be used or relied on, in whole or in part, for the diagnosis or treatment of any physical, emotional, and/or psychological condition of any type or nature for persons in the twenty-first century.

A Note on Language

Some of the settings and language in the book portray women in a submissive role within their family and in society. The book was written twenty-two years prior to the enactment of the nineteenth amendment to the constitution of the United States on August 20, 1920. The amendment recognized the right of American women to vote, furthering equality for women in the United States. We hope for more progress in women's rights and equal treatment under the law.

Introduction

Every mother desires that her children shall be strong and well. She does not always realize that the responsibility of making and keeping them so belongs in large measure to her. She regulates their food, their clothing and, to a great extent, their surroundings; it is on these that their health depends.

Often, while earnestly desiring to do what is best for them, she fails from want of knowledge of what is best.

It is well known, for example, that children cannot grow and develop properly without suitable, nutritious food. This is not always what is proper for older persons, nor what a child would take from choice. It must be palatable enough to be relished, or it will not be eaten in sufficient quantities; it must contain the elements that are necessary to build up muscles, nerves and bones, or the body suffers.

If the mother does not know the kinds of food that will best serve these ends, she is depriving her children of proper nourishment, although it may seem to her they have more than enough to eat.

The care of children has never received as much attention as is being given to it at the present time. The wise mother will try to keep abreast of modern thought in this matter and to take advantage of the experience of others for her children's good.

A year or two ago the writer, in her capacity as editor of the "Mother's Corner" of "The Ladies' Home Journal," received between twelve and thirteen hundred letters asking for advice as to the care of infants. In response to these requests a pamphlet was written called "A Baby's Requirements."

Elizabeth Robinson Scovil *The Care of Children*

This pamphlet brought forth so many inquiries as to the care of children after babyhood that it was determined to expand it into a larger volume, containing, beside the greater part of the original matter, the information desired.

An experience of many years in hospital work has given a familiarity with the details of nursing that it is hoped will render the chapters on the care of illness especially useful. It is then that the inexperienced mother most feels her helplessness and welcomes friendly aid.

In many childish ailments the nursing equals in importance the medical treatment. Sometimes the knowledge of what ought to be done in the beginning is all-important and makes no slight difference in the result.

An effort has been made in *The Care of Children* to answer in a plain and practical manner the questions that are most likely to arise to puzzle those to whom this charge is entrusted, whether in sickness or in health.

If the book is a help to mothers – experienced or inexperienced – in their moments of perplexity, its existence will be amply justified.

Table of Contents

PHYSICAL DEFORMITIES — 135

The Care of Children

FOOD
CHAPTER I

NURSING

It is impossible for a child to grow and thrive unless it has suitable food. Most of the disorders of young children, particularly babies, arise from errors in diet. Either the kind of food or the quantity given is in fault.

If a mother can nurse her child, the problem of nourishing it is usually an easy one to solve. Sometimes, however, even the mother's milk does not agree with the baby, and then, unless she can alter it by dieting herself, a substitute must be found for it.

The first fluid secreted by the breast is a thin liquid called colostrum. This acts as a cathartic and relieves the child of an accumulation of waste matter, the meconium.

The colostrum is not very nutritious, but it is all that nature provides for the baby until it is about two days old, and she seldom makes mistakes. If for any reason the child cannot be nursed, it needs very little food until the third day.

In nursing, the baby should be held comfortably on the mother's arm, the breast being pressed back a little with the finger that it may not obstruct the nostrils, as the child has to breathe through the nose. If the milk comes too quickly, it can be checked by gentle pressure with the fingers.

The baby should nurse from either side alternately, having one at each nursing.

If any preparation has been used on the nipple, it should be carefully washed before the baby takes it. After withdrawing it, bathe it again in warm water and gently wash out the child's mouth with a little swab, made of a piece of fine handkerchief, dipped in cool water. If these precautions are neglected, the particles of milk decompose and give rise to a fungoid growth called thrush, which may be fatal to a young baby.

Should this happen through carelessness, put a pinch of borax in a couple of tablespoons full of water and wash the mouth with it frequently.

When the coming of milk is delayed, or the baby is an exceptionally vigorous child, it grows very hungry, and, not getting enough from the breast to satisfy it, protests loudly against this condition of affairs. During the first two days a few teaspoons of warm water may be tried. If this does not meet the requirements, mix two teaspoonfuls of cow's milk with four of boiled water and add a very little sugar of milk to sweeten it. The latter can be procured of any druggist. It is a powder and very inexpensive.

INTERVALS OF NURSING

This amount of food can be given not oftener than every four hours, putting the child to the breast once between each feeding.

If the mother is comfortable, the baby should try to nurse first about four hours after it is born, and then at the same interval for the first two days.

After that it should be nursed once in two hours during the day and six at night.

A baby soon learns good habits if it is fairly dealt with, and it is very important that it should not be disturbed at night.

No child wants food every time it cries. There are other causes for the discomfort that it can only express in one way.

If it is fed too often the stomach cannot dispose of the quantity of food forced into it. If it does manage to digest it there are grumbles of discontent at the overwork, which the mother too often interprets as a demand for more food. Fortunately, babies vomit easily and so get rid of the surplus, but it is better not to overtax their limited capacity.

Usually, a baby requires to nurse about ten or fifteen minutes. When satisfied, it will leave off of its own accord and drop asleep.

Milk, which requires two hours to digest in the stomach of an adult, is disposed of by a baby's digestive apparatus in about half the time. Thus, feeding every two hours allows a sufficient interval of rest.

CARE OF THE BREASTS

It is very important for the mother's future comfort that the breasts should be properly attended to before the birth of the child. They enlarge and are usually more or less sensitive. No pressure upon them should be permitted, a comfortably fitting waist being worn instead of corsets.

Dissolve a little salt in brandy, or a pinch of alum in alcohol, and bathe the nipples with it every night for six weeks, pressing and pulling them gently at the same time.

Dr. Starr recommends bathing them in warm water in the evening and anointing them with cocoa butter in the morning. Both processes have given good results. Probably a thin, delicate skin would be more benefited by the first, and a thicker, tougher one by the last mentioned.

Elizabeth Robinson Scovil *The Care of Children*

If the nipple is retracted, or pushed inward, fill a pint bottle with hot water, empty it quickly and place the mouth of the bottle over the nipple. As the air in it cools the nipple will be drawn out and can then be taken between the fingers and manipulated.

When there has been no preparation, the first efforts of the baby to nurse may cause the skin of the nipple to crack and it becomes very sore, so much so, that nursing may have to be abandoned on this account alone.

At the first suspicious symptom, white of egg should be painted on the sensitive surface, making two or three applications and letting it dry. If this does not succeed, a pinch of powdered tannic acid can be stirred into glycerin and applied after each nursing, being washed off with a solution of boracic acid before the child nurses again.

A rubber nipple-shield should be provided to cover that of the mother while the child is nursing. Glass shields are sold, which can be worn in the interval and make the part more comfortable.

If the breast is hard, or contains lumps, it should be *very gently* but persistently rubbed from the base towards the nipple until it is soft. Neglect of this measure may result in an abscess.

When for any cause the milk has to be dried up, the doctor will order a lotion ointment, or plaster, for the purpose.

When the breasts feel heavy and uncomfortable, they should be supported with a bandage shaped like the letter Y. The straight piece goes across the back, being made about twice as long as is needed. One side of the fork of the Y goes above the breasts, the other below them, and the points are pinned to the long piece. The extra length is brought over the nipples and can easily be turned back without disturbing the bandage when the child is to be nursed. Absorbent cotton can be put between the breasts and about them, under the bandage.

To make it, take two strips of cotton three inches wide and a yard long. Fold one in the middle so that the two ends come at an acute angle, and fasten it with safety-pins to the end of the straight strip. If it is not secure after it is in place, it can be fastened with straps over the shoulders.

The mother should always have a light shawl, or other covering, thrown over the breast when the baby is nursing.

When the Milk Discharges

Sometimes the mother's milk is insufficient in quantity, or not rich enough to satisfy the child. When this is the case, it must be nursed once in four hours and fed between each nursing.

The mother can drink milk, cocoa, albuminized milk; that is, the white of one egg to each half pint of milk, shaken in a self-sealing glass jar, or bottle, and gruel of oatmeal, Indian meal, or barley made with milk. Plenty of fluid increases the flow of milk. The breast can be gently rubbed from the base of the nipple twice a day with warm camphorated oil, and the child encouraged to nurse. The act of sucking stimulates the secretion of milk. As much nourishing food as possible should be taken, good soup, meat and fresh vegetables, as well as the cereals. This helps to improve the quality of the milk.

When the baby does not digest its food properly it cries with pain after nursing, or throws up the milk curdled, or sour, and there are white curds of milk in the motions. It is restless and fretful, and the skin may be hotter than usual.

Two teaspoonfuls of lime water given just before nursing will sometimes obviate the difficulty, and one or two may follow the meal.

The doctor may have to prescribe if the case is obstinate. Medicine should not be given without her prescription.

Something in the mother's diet may not agree with the delicate stomach of the child. Acids are apt to affect it unpleasantly — as vinegar, or sour fruits, as strawberries, and occasionally vegetables, as tomatoes. Only experience can show what must be avoided. Articles that will not affect one baby may cause another much discomfort.

The possibility of the child being overfed should always be borne in mind. When the stomach feels hard and distended, or the milk is vomited soon after being swallowed, looking unchanged, the child should be kept at the breast a shorter time for the next meal.

If the child is being properly nourished it will gain steadily in weight. It loses during the first three days, but after that gains about three-quarters of a pound or more during the first month. During the second month it should increase in weight from a quarter to half a pound each week: after that the gain is more slow, but should progress constantly until at six months old it gains about a pound a month. The increase is often more rapid, but this proportion shows that the baby is thriving.

Elizabeth Robinson Scovil *The Care of Children*

When Nursing is Improper

It is the duty and ought to be the pleasure of every mother to nurse her own baby. All right-thinking women are anxious to do so in spite of the inconvenience to themselves. Yet there are cases in which this privilege must be denied.

If the mother is afflicted with a constitutional disease, as scrofula or consumption, her milk will be injurious to the baby. Should there be a return of the menstrual flow nursing must be discontinued. Some women have not sufficient strength to nourish their children without injuring their own health, but no one should hastily decide that this is the case.

If the milk manifestly disagrees with the baby its use cannot be continued. This is shown by the child losing flesh and becoming pale and puny. A well-nourished infant has firm flesh, slightly mottled, a good color in the lips, and bright, clear eyes.

Weaning

When the mother has been happy enough to be able to nurse her baby, she is apt to prolong the pleasure beyond due limits. No child should be nursed after it is a year old, and there are many reasons that may make it necessary to withdraw the natural nourishment much earlier.

One has to be mentioned: its insufficiency to meet the demands of the child.

Very often the supply of milk diminishes, the breasts do not fill, and it is evident there is not enough to satisfy the hungry applicant.

Sometimes the mother's health suffers; she feels languid and miserable, grows thin, has constant headache and no appetite. She has pain between the shoulders and is always tired. The drain upon her vitality is too great and she cannot do justice to the child.

When the weaning can be done gradually, there is usually little discomfort on either side. If the baby has a food that it likes, alternately with the breasts, for the first day or two, it will not rebel. It can be given more often each day, at the time the child has been accustomed to be nursed, until finally it is substituted entirely, and the weaning is accomplished.

The process is more painful, to the mother at least, when, for any cause, it has to be done suddenly and there is an abundance of milk.

The breasts should be comfortably supported with a bandage, and a handkerchief, wrung out of alcohol diluted with an equal quantity of water, laid on them and kept wet. Very little liquid should be drunk and a gentle laxative taken; a heaping teaspoonful of Epson or Rochelle salts, citrate of magnesia, or a Seidlitz powder.

Sometimes the breasts are rubbed with belladonna liniment, or painted with a mixture of belladonna and glycerin; or a belladonna plaster, cut round, with a hole in the middle for the nipple, is applied.

When there is an unusual quantity of milk, it may have to be drawn with a breast pump. This should be avoided if possible, as it tends to keep up the secretion instead of checking it. If a baby is thriving it is best not to wean it in summer, as a change of food may disagree with it and cause diarrhea, which is to be dreaded in warm weather.

Teething need not be an obstacle to weaning, unless the child suffers very much and is made ill by the process, when it is unwise to add to its troubles by any experiment in new diet, unless the breast milk disagrees with it.

Elizabeth Robinson Scovil *The Care of Children*

CHAPTER II

FEEDING

When a baby cannot be nursed, life depends upon a food being found which it can digest.

Cows' milk is the one most easily obtained and when properly prepared makes the best substitute. It contains less sugar of milk and fat than that of a human mother and these must be supplied — the fat by adding cream to it. It is slightly acid, instead of being alkaline; this can be corrected by the addition of lime water. There is more caseine, or the hard curd of which cheese is made, than in mothers' milk, and water must be added to reduce this.

These points are all covered in a recipe prepared by Dr. Meigs, called:

CREAM FOOD

Cream, 2 tablespoonfuls.
Milk, 1 tablespoonful.
Lime water, 2 tablespoonfuls.
Milk-sugar water, 3 tablespoonfuls.

One-quarter of this quantity can be given every two hours during the day and once or twice at night, if necessary, until the baby is a week old.

After that the quantity must be increased, one-half the amount prepared being given at once, until at two months old and the child takes the whole quantity. The proportion of milk is gradually increased and the water lessened, the cream also being decreased, until when two months old the baby is taking:

Milk, 3 tablespoonfuls.
Cream, 1 tablespoonful.
Lime water, 1 tablespoonful.
Sugar water, 3 tablespoonfuls.

After two months the lime water may be discontinued and the milk gradually increased, until at five months old the child has five tablespoonfuls of milk instead of three, the cream and sugar water remaining unchanged.

When it is six months old the quantity of milk is doubled; that is, increased every day until it has ten tablespoonfuls at each feeding.

The milk used for a baby should be allowed to stand in a cool place for three hours after being received to allow the cream to rise. The upper half is then carefully dipped off with a saucer or ladle and the remainder set aside for other uses. The baby must have the best.

MILK SUGAR WATER
To make this, dissolve half an ounce of sugar of milk in a half pint of boiling water. It will not keep long after it is made.

LIME WATER
This is expensive if bought and is easily prepared at home at the most trifling cost. Take a lump of lime as large as a good-sized plum — it weighs about an ounce. Put it in a bottle with one quart of cold water which has previously been boiled. Shake the bottle well until the lime is dissolved and let it stand for twelve hours before using. Pour it carefully into another bottle so as not to disturb the sediment. Water can only absorb a certain quantity of lime, about a quarter of a grain to a tablespoonful, so there is no fear of it being too strong.

BARLEY FOOD
As cows' milk forms firmer curds in the stomach of a baby than its mother's milk would do, it is sometimes impossible for this delicate organ to break them up and digest them. Barley seems to have the power of remedying this defect and barley food may be tried when the milk and lime water disagree with the baby.

To make it, take two even tablespoonfuls of pearl barley. After washing it thoroughly put it in a double boiler, or saucepan, with one pint of boiling water and let it boil two hours. Ground barley need only be cooked half an hour. Use the barley water instead of the lime water and sugar water in the cream food and sweeten with a tiny pinch of dry sugar of milk.

MALTED FOOD
Dr. H. D. Chapin and Dr. Arnold Eiloart, of New York, have been carrying out a series of experiments to ascertain a cheap and satisfactory method of preparing an easily digested food for babies. Their formula is given with the permission of the former:

> Wheat flour, or barley meal, two ounces; that is, 2 tablespoon-
> fuls heaped as high as possible.
> Water, fifty-six ounces, or a quart and three-quarters.

Elizabeth Robinson Scovil *The Care of Children*

Extract of malt, a small teaspoonful.

Mix the flour to a paste with the little water, gradually thinned this with a scant quart of water, put it into a double boiler and boil it 10 minutes. Take out the inner vessel and add the rest of the water cold, the malt extract being dissolved in the last few tables tablespoons full. Let it stand 15 minutes. Put back the inner vessel in the double boiler, and heat again 15 minutes. Strain through a wire gauze strainer.

Half the quantity may be made, using pints instead of quarts and measuring the water.

This preparation is used instead of barley water, lime water or sugar water and diluting the milk. It should not, of course, be given without milk.

In making the gruel, it must be stirred while cooking until it thickens or it will not be smooth. In the outer part of the double boiler must boil all the time.

The malted water enriches the milk and prevents it from coagulating into the large, tough curds that are so objectionable in the baby's stomach.

Peptonized Milk

If the baby's digestion is seriously affected it may be necessary partially to digest the milk before giving it. This process is known as peptonizing it.

Extract of pancreas can be obtained from the druggist, Five grains of this and fifteen grains of the baking soda are added to each pint of milk.

Tablets of pancreatin and soda can also be used.

After adding the peptonizing agent place the milk in water at of a temperature of 115°F, or so hot that the hand can be dipped in water only for a moment. Leave it there for 20 minutes and then place it on the ice, or pour the milk into a clean saucepan and bring it to the boil, to stop the digestive process. If this is carried the least too far the milk will taste bitter. It is well to try it from time to time and if any change is detected to take it out of the hot water at once.

Either cream food or barley food can be peptonized. This pre-digestion has undoubtedly saved the lives of many children who are unable to digest food for themselves. The use of peptonized food should only be continued until the child gains strength, as it is not well to interfere with the natural process too long.

Sterilized Milk

Milk is a frequent carrier of infection and in cities particularly it is very difficult to get it perfectly pure.

Sterilizing destroys any germs that may contain and renders it a safer food for the baby.

It was once thought necessary to boil it, but it is now said that if the milk is heated to a temperature of 180° Fahrenheit and kept at this point for fifteen minutes, it will keep for twenty-four hours, and the flavor of the milk is not injured as by boiling. Water boils at 212°F, so this is some distance below the boiling point.

Probably the easiest and most practical way for the mother to manage this important business is to provide six to eight half-pint bottles, according to the number of times the child is fed in twenty-four hours. Put the proper amount of food for one feeding in each bottle and use a tuft of cotton batting as a stopper.

Have a saucepan that the bottles can stand in conveniently. Invert a perforated tin pie plate in the bottom and put in enough water to come well above the milk in the bottles. Stand the bottles on it and when the water boils draw the saucepan to a cooler part of the stove. Cover the saucepan and let the bottles remain in the hot water one hour. Then put them in the ice box or stand them in cold water, or a cool place in winter.

In sterilizing milk to use on a long journey repeat the process three times, letting the milk cool between each.

Patent sterilizers can be bought and are very convenient, but the home utensils answer every purpose.

It is worthwhile for the mother to take the trouble to be certain that her baby is having pure milk. Unless she draws it from the cow herself, or is *sure* of the conditions under which it is drawn, it is wisest to sterilize it.

It is said that if a wad of cotton batting is placed in a funnel, the cold milk poured on it and allowed to filter slowly through into a pitcher, many impurities are strained out of it. The fibers of the cotton have the power of arresting germs and the proportion is much smaller in the filtered milk. This experiment is worth trying when for any reason it is impossible to sterilize the milk by heat.

Condensed Milk

Condensed milk, sold in tins, is not a suitable food for a baby. It contains a large quantity of sugar, which makes the child fat, but not enough material to build up the muscles and form firm flesh. It is a laxative, and when there is constipation one meal daily may be given of it to secure the desired result. It would not injure a child to be fed on it for two or three days, as in travelling, when it is difficult to procure fresh milk; but it's use should not be long continued.

A baby's food must contain the elements necessary to build up the different parts of the body and fresh milk is the only one that combines all of these.

One teaspoonful of condensed milk to one cup, or eight tablespoonfuls, of water is about the right proportion. If it is necessary to use it for any length of time, it is well to add one teaspoonful of cream.

Always put a little salt in baby's food.

AMOUNT OF FOOD

A baby's stomach at the time of birth is said to hold about six teaspoonfuls, so that at first it needs very little food at a time. The capacity increases rapidly during the first and second months and not so fast from the third to the fifth.

A child who has come into the world prematurely may not be able to take more than a few drops of nourishment at a time, and these have to be administered with a medicine dropper. There is no strength to suck and no power to assimilate a quantity of food.

Many authorities maintained that the amount of a child's food should be regulated by its weight rather than wholly by its age, a child of from six to eight pounds requiring after the first week about six tablespoonfuls at a feeding once in two hours from 6:00 AM to 8:00 PM and once during the night. The amount is gradually increased and the interval lengthened until the child weighing twenty pounds has sixteen tablespoonfuls every three hours during the day, and once at night if necessary.

Children should have food as often as once in three hours during the day until they are four years old; that is, a glass of milk, or some simple nourishment, between breakfast and dinner and dinner and tea.

The appetite varies even in babies, some infants requiring more food than others. It may be necessary to feed a child every hour and a half if it wakes and is manifestly hungry, but the feeding should be delayed if possible. On the other hand, some babies seem not to need food so often and will accept very contentedly a meal once in three hours.

Each baby must be judged on its own merits; it is only possible to lay down general principles for the treatment. Common sense must guide the application.

TEMPERATURE OF FOOD

Too hot food is a fruitful source of trouble with young babies. It should never be more than "milk warm," about 99°F, as this is nearly the temperature of its natural food.

Heating Food

If the baby is fed once during the night, it is convenient to warm the milk in the bottle before the mother goes to bed and wrap it in a blanket within easy reach. It will be about the right heat in four or five hours, when it is needed. It's still too warm let it stand uncovered for a few moments.

If it has been sterilized it will not be injured by waiting. In summer, or when the nursery is at a distance from the kitchen, it is convenient to have a small saucepan for warming the food. This can be filled with water to stand the bottle in and heated in a few minutes.

Tin chimneys with a mica slide in the side can be obtained that will fit a kerosene lamp, or little contrivances to put over a gas burner, either of which will support a saucepan.

The Nursing Bottle

Provide two plain round bottles, as they are the most easily kept clean, and half a dozen rubber tops without tubes. Graduated bottles with ounces or tablespoonfuls marked on the outside can be purchased and make it easier to measure the exact quantity of food.

After using, empty any milk that may be left in it; rinse in cool water, then in scalding water and turned it up to dry. If particles of milk adhere to the bottle, use coarse salt, or raw potato cut in small pieces, to remove them. If the bottle looks clouded, add a little ammonia to the water, rinsing the bottle of thoroughly in clear water.

The rubber tops should be turned inside out and scrubbed with a stiff brush kept for the purpose. Once in two or three days they should be boiled for ten minutes.

The most delicate cleanliness is absolutely necessary in the care of the bottle and the top. The want of it will surely cause serious illness to the child.

As soon as possible a baby should be taught to drink from a cup and the nursing bottle abandoned.

Giving the Food

The mother must not grudge the time that is necessary to feed her baby. The child should be placed in a comfortable position and its crib and the mother sit by it and hold the bottle at such an angle that the top is kept filled with milk.

If the bottle is laid on its side air is sucked in with the milk and a stomach-ache may result. After a meal the baby should lie on its right side. The liver is disproportionately large in young children and if it presses on the stomach digestion is interfered with.

When the child sleeps after eating, in about an hour it should be gently turned on the left side. It is not well for it to lie always in one position, as in time this may cause deformity.

Water

Water is very necessary for children. They often cry from thirst instead of hunger. A young baby should have a teaspoon full several times a day and the quantity be increased as it grows older. The lack of sufficient water with the food is a frequent cause of constipation.

If there is any reason to suspect its purity it should be boiled. The flat taste that boiling gives it can be removed by shaking it in the jar, or pitcher, so it can regain the oxygen, of which boiling deprived it.

CHAPTER III

INCREASING THE FOOD

After a food has been found that agrees with the baby it usually thrives well upon it; the quantity being increased as the child grows older. When the first teeth are through, or it is about six to seven months old, it may begin to seem dissatisfied with milk alone and to demand an addition to its diet. What this is to be is an important question, and often several kinds of food have to be tried before the right one is chosen.

A young baby cannot digest food containing a large amount of starch. Saliva is necessary to convert this into sugar, and there is no secretion of saliva in a baby's mouth before it is four months old. For some time starchy food must be given very sparingly.

Arrowroot is out of the question because it is chiefly composed of starch. Barley gruel, which has already been spoken of, and oatmeal gruel, make a suitable addition. It must be borne in mind that the gruels are only added; the chief reliance must still be placed on milk.

Oatmeal Gruel

A delicate gruel can be made by rolling a cup of oatmeal on a cake board, or pounding it with a pestle. Put this in a dish and pour over it about a pint of water. Stir it up, and let the mixture settle for a minute. Pour off the milky fluid and repeat the process twice. Boil this water for an hour, adding a little salt, and use it to dilute the milk instead of water.

Gruel can be made from oatmeal by allowing one tablespoonful to each cup of boiling water, boiling one hour and straining through a wire strainer.

Farina Gruel

Farina is prepared from the most nutritious part of the wheat. Being already partially cooked, it does not require as long boiling as the other cereals. Take one tablespoonful of farina the two cups of boiling water, add salt, and cook for fifteen minutes. Use as directed for oatmeal gruel.

Flour Ball

This may be given to babies under four months old, as the long boiling converts the starch into dextrin, a substance between starch and grape sugar, and digestible by young children. It is especially recommended in cases of diarrhea and may be used instead of barley gruel as a food.

To make it, put a bowl full of flour into a stout cloth, tie it up like a pudding, put it in a sauce pan of boiling water, and boil it for ten or twelve hours. On removing, turn it out of the cloth and cut away the soft outside. When cool, grate the hard inside portion and use one teaspoonful at each feeding for a baby eight months old, increasing the amount for an older child.

Rice Water

This is valuable as a food during diarrhea, or when for any cause the use of milk has to be discontinued for a time.

Wash two tablespoonfuls of rice and put it in a quart of boiling, salted water. Let it cook for two hours, until the rice is nearly dissolved. Pour the liquid through a strainer, or a piece of thin muslin, and give it to cool.

Whey Food

Mix one teaspoonful of liquid rennet with one pint of milk. Set it in a warm place, but not where it will become more than milk-warm. When the curd forms, break it up with a spoon, beating it well, and strain off the whey. This can be given alone when milk cannot be digested, or with one quarter part cream added to it.

Albuminized Food

Shake the white of an egg with half a pint of water and a self-sealing glass jar until they are thoroughly mixed. Add two grains of salt. It may be given alone when milk cannot be taken, or with the addition of one-third milk or one-fourth cream.

Beef Juice

When the four front teeth are through, or after the child is nine months old, it may have once a day one or two tablespoonfuls of beef juice, not beef tea. This may be the juice that runs from rare roast beef when it is cut, or it may be specially prepared for the purpose. In this case cut half a pound of steak for the top of the round into pieces about one inch square. Place them in a glass jar or bottle, stand this in cold water over the fire. Let the water heat gradually until it is scalding hot, but not boiling, about 180°F, and keep it at this temperature one hour. Then pour out the juice and add a little salt for use.

Mutton can be treated in the same way.

The juice can be pressed from the rare meat with a lemon squeezer, the steak bean first broiled for a minute, but it is a more troublesome process and not as much is obtained.

This addition to the diet often relieves constipation.

It should be remembered that young children do not require a great variety in their food. A baby who is nursed by its mother has only her milk until it is at least ten months old.

When the teeth are well developed, it is nature's indication that the little body is ready to digest and assimilate more solid food than milk. The wise mother gives it, but only one new article of diet at a time, and waits to see how it is disposed of before introducing another novelty.

After the child is a year old, the cereals, instead of being made into gruel, can be eaten as porridge with a little sugar. Hominy, cracked wheat, and farinose may be added to the list, and, a little later, rice. All the cereals should be thoroughly cooked.

BREAD

Almost all children like bread and milk, and most babies make their first attempt at masticating solid food with a crust of bread. This is rather a dangerous plaything, as they are apt to bite off a piece which they cannot swallow with ease. Finely crumbled, or softened with warm milk, it is a very desirable form of food.

Bread for babies, or young children, should be at least one day old. Chewing fresh bread converts it into a pasty which the saliva cannot penetrate to digest the starch. It passes into the stomach, where it cannot be dealt with, and is a source of irritation there. Milk toast, made by pouring hot milk over thin slices of well toasted bread, is unobjectionable.

CRACKERS

Gluten, soda, oatmeal and Graham crackers can be given, at first soaked in milk and later alone. These are better than the square, sweet biscuit in which children usually delight.

EGGS

A properly cooked egg is easily digested by a child a year old, and one every day, or every other day, may be given.

When an egg is plunged into boiling water and cooked for three or four minutes, the albuminous part, or white, is hardened into a tough, solid mass, difficult for the digestive powers of an adult to deal with.

Pour a pint of boiling water into a saucepan, put in the egg, leaving the vessel uncovered, and draw it to a cool part of the stove where the water will not boil again. In ten minutes the egg will be done, the white bean like a soft Jelly instead of hard leather.

The egg may be poached by breaking it carefully into a saucer and sliding it into a saucepan of boiling, salted water. Do not let the water boil after it is in and cook it two minutes.

SCRAMBLED EGG

An egg may be beaten with two tablespoonsful of milk and stirred in a hot frying- pan over a moderate fire, drawing it aside every few seconds so that the mass will not cook too quickly and be soft and light when done. If there is whey it has remained on the fire too long, and the hard curds should not be given to the child.

Fried eggs are indigestible and must be prohibited.

STIRRED EGG

The yoke of an egg can be put in a cup and set in boiling water and stirred until it thickens. Add a little salt.

JUNKET

Junket is also called curds and rennet custard. It is the albuminous, or flesh-forming part of milk separated into a curd by the addition of rennet. Liquid rennet can be bought from the grocer or druggist and is extracted from the inner lining of the stomach of the calf.

Junket is much better for children of a year old, and upwards, than custard or puddings, and may be tried for babies who object to milk in a fluid form.

To make it, take one pint of milk, warm it to 98°F, or milk-warm, add one teaspoon of rennet and one teaspoonful of sugar; stir all together and let it stand in a warm place until it sets, or becomes semi-solid. Remove it to a cold place or the coagulation will go too far and whey will appear.

BAKED POTATO

This is the only form in which potato should be given to a child under two years old. The potash salts, which are a valuable constituent of the potato, are lost when it is peeled and boiled; while the skin retains them during baking. It should be perfectly cooked, dry and mealy, and be given with little salt and a dessert's spoonful of cream rather than butter.

GELATINE CREAM

Put one-quarter of the box of gelatin in a quarter of a cup of cold water; let it soak for half an hour, then set the bowl on top of a boiling tea kettle or in hot water and stir until the gelatin is dissolved.

Pour it into a cold dish and when it begins to stiffen add one and a half cups of good milk, or half cream and half milk, a teaspoon of sugar, a little cinnamon, lemon juice, or vanilla, if desired.

MACARONI

Being made from wheat flour, either macaroni or vermicelli is excellent for children. It should be dropped into boiling milk, or half milk and half water, and heat lost by putting in a cold macaroni being restored by adding a little boiling water. If this is not done it will be pasty from soaking in the cooled water. Boil until tender, adding a little salt.

RICE

This is an excellent food for children and can be cooked in a variety of ways. When done, each grain should be distinct yet soft.

To boil it, put half a cup of well washed rice in one quarter boiling water, adding a little boiling water to keep up the heat and a good pinch of salt. It will cook in from fifteen to twenty minutes and must be removed while the water is perfectly clear. If the grains burst the starch gives the water a milky appearance. Drain the rice and return it to the saucepan to dry for a minute, stirring it lightly with a fork.

To steam it in a boat double boiler, use one cup of boiling water in half a cup of rice that has been thoroughly washed. Add a little salt and cook for half an hour. Remove the cover and let the rice dry. Milk can be used instead of water or half of each. Chicken or beef broth can be substituted for the milk or water, for children requiring especially nourishing food.

Stirred Rice — Put half a teaspoon of rice in one quart of milk, sweeten to taste and bake slowly until the milk is absorbed, stirring frequently. If the milk boils away pour in a little more from time to time. When done the pudding should be a soft creamy mass.

Eggs may be added to rice pudding and cinnamon, lemon, vanilla, rose water, or any flavoring desired.

Elizabeth Robinson Scovil *The Care of Children*

ORANGES

The year-old baby may have the juice of half an orange and, as he grows older, the pulp scraped from its covering membrane and divested of the seeds. The orange juice should be given midway between the meals of milk as they sometimes disagree if brought into too close contact.

Orange juice given early in the morning is an excellent laxative. For this reason, neither it nor apple should be given when there is a tendency to diarrhea.

BAKED APPLES

The baby will enjoy the soft part of a baked apple when he has passed his first birthday. Very little sugar should be given with it. It is never well to begin the use of fruit in very warm weather. If the child has become accustomed to taking it, its use need not be discontinued unless it disagrees with him.

Other fruit and vegetables should not be given until after the child is two years old.

CHAPTER IV

DIET AFTER TWO YEARS OF AGE

MEAT

It is stated that children from two to four years of age require about one-fourth as much food as a grown person at the active, working age. There is a large amount of tissue to be built up and the proper supply of suitable food is very important. It is a mistaken idea that children require a quantity of meat, to strengthen them, as it is said.

Nutritious food is that which gives to the body the different substances it needs to build up its various parts. Meat feeds the muscles but does not develop bone. The salts necessary for this purpose must be supplied by vegetables, including in this term cereals and fruits.

Meat stimulates the nervous system and increases the activity of the brain, so that its use should be restricted in the case of nervous children.

When taken in excess it is said to render the disposition irritable and quarrelsome; and that children whose diet it predominates do not grow as tall as those fed on less stimulating fare.

Until the full set of first teeth have come, which usually occurs between twenty months and two years and a half old, a child should not have meat, except in the form of meat juice, broth or soup. After that it can be given in small quantities once a day, never more often.

Its place should be supplied by an abundance of milk. Bread, porridge of the various cereals, eggs, delicate vegetables, and fruit constituting the remainder of the diet.

COOKING MEAT

In giving meat to a child and cooking is a matter of prime importance. The albumen it contains can be hardened just as the white of an egg is by improper cooking.

Children should be encouraged to like rare meat. If there is a distaste for it, this can sometimes be overcome by giving it a little less well done each day. As long as it looks red it is sufficiently rare for practical purposes.

Roast beef, mutton, or chicken are suitable for children. Veal, pork and salt meat, as ham, and the internal organs, liver, kidneys, sweetbreads, etc., must be avoided.

Elizabeth Robinson Scovil *The Care of Children*

Meat should be either roasted or broiled, although boiled chicken and mutton are permissible. Frying, as it is usually done, renders meat unfit for human digestion.

It should not be chosen as a means of cooking meat for children, but if it cannot be avoided, heat the frying pan hot, putting in a small piece of dripping, and when it melts, the meat, turning the ladder quickly from side to side. Use as little fat as possible and remove the meat the instant it is sufficiently done.

BEEF STEAK

Have the hot fire, place the steak on the gridiron and hold it close to the fire for a minute, turning it rapidly. The fierce heat coagulates the albumen near the surface, seals the pores of the meat and keeps in the juice. When the outside is seared, hold it farther from the fire until it is done. On removing, sprinkle it with salt.

Steak should be cut about one inch thick. The top of the round is a juicy and well flavored part of the beef, and steak cut from there is less expensive than the sirloin, or choicer steaks, and more nutritious.

MUTTON CHOPS

These are cooked in the same way as beef steak. They should be nicely trimmed, and the fat removed before broiling.

SOUPS

When meat is to be made into soup it should be cut in pieces, the bones broken, and placed in cold water, which is gradually heated, to draw out the juices.

In cooking meat, intended to be eaten, it should be plunged into boiling water to seal the pores and keep the juices in.

CHICKEN

Poultry is not more desirable for children than beef or mutton, although, being more delicate, it is sometimes considered so. Either the white or dark meat may be given, the former being preferable. It may be roasted, boiled or broiled.

BACON

Fat is essential to the proper growth of the tissues of the nerves and the brain, and is peculiarly important to children, as the brain enlarges rapidly during childhood. Next to butter and cream, bacon is one of the most palatable forms in which it can be given. It should not be overcooked, as then too much of the fat is fried out. Sometimes bread soaked in bacon fat will be eaten with relish.

Salt pork, well soaked, thoroughly boiled, cut in thin slices and eaten as a sandwich between thin slices of bread, makes a good substitute or alternative.

VEGETABLES

After a child is two years old a vegetable of some kind beside potato may be given at midday meal. Cabbage, raw cucumbers, and green corn are unsuitable, but any other well-cooked vegetable is harmless in small quantities. Stewed celery, peas, beans, tender cauliflower, baked or stewed tomato are all useful.

FRUIT

Any fresh, ripe, seasonable fruit may be given early in the day to a child who is well. The points to observe are to have it sound; that is, without a suspicion of staleness, and not to give too much at once. Strawberries, raspberries, blackberries, pears, apples, peaches, oranges and grapes are all welcome.

Fruit having a skin should be pared, and grapes should have the seeds removed, or the child should be taught not to swallow them.

Bananas must be given with caution; they disagree with many children. Try a slice one day and, if no ill effects follow, to the next, proceeding slowly until certain it can be well borne.

STEWED FRUIT

Stewed fruit can be given at supper and is much relished by most children.

Apples, pears and peaches cooked in this way are valuable addition to the diet list, and almost any of the fresh fruits can be similarly treated.

In winter evaporated apples, apricots, nectarines, etc., are nearly as nice as the fresh fruit and bear little resemblance to the old fashioned, leather-like dried preparations. They must be soaked overnight before cooking and boiled until perfectly tender.

Prunes with the stones removed are a favorite dish in many nurseries.

The craving which children have for sweet things indicates a legitimate demand for sugar, which should be met by giving sweets at meals with other food, instead of allowing unlimited indulgence in candy between times.

Bread and molasses, or syrup, or maple syrup may be safely eaten when chocolate creams or caramels would cause a fit of indigestion

Elizabeth Robinson Scovil *The Care of Children*

PUDDINGS

No young child should taste pastry. After seven years of age a little may be given occasionally if it is light, flaky and well baked.

Its place can be filled with advantage by puddings of rice, tapioca, corn starch, baked Indian meal, sago, baked and boiled custard, and all the varieties of blanc mange and creams that can be made with corn starch or gelatin, milk and eggs.

Ice cream is beneficial to children if it is not given in too large quantity.

Rice puddings should be avoided just as rich-made dishes are, because the simpler the food the stomach has to deal with the better.

BEVERAGES

A child, until it is twelve years old, should drink little beside milk or water. Tea and coffee are stimulants and are better left untouched by a nervous race like ourselves, as long as possible.

Milk can be diluted with hot water if necessary, and sweetened, when it is called "cambric tea."

Children who do not care for milk can sometimes be induced to take it by adding a few drops of vanilla and a little sugar and calling it "ice cream milk" or by boiling part of the rind of a lemon in it with sugar. Sometimes merely heating it will overcome the distaste for cold milk and a pinch of salt may be added. Cocoa, cocoa nibs, or chocolate are good for children from the quantity of fat they contain. They should be made with half milk and half water.

Ice water is injurious to the delicate stomach of a child. The water can be cooled by keeping it in a stoneware pitcher in the ice chest. When no ice is at hand, wrap the pitcher in a wet cloth and standing in a draught, changing the cloth once or twice as it dries. The heat is removed by evaporation.

A small quantity of home-made fruit syrup may be added to it as a treat.

FRUIT SYRUP

To make this, take two quarts of strawberries or raspberries and two pounds of sugar, put them in a jar standing in boiling water, and let them remain for an hour. This draws the juice out. Turn the contents of the jar into a wire sieve placed over a large bowl and let the juice drain off without pressing the fruit. Have ready some self-sealing jars, scalded with boiling water, fill these with the juice, stand them in a saucepan of cold water over the fire and let them remain in it half an hour after the water boils; screw on the tops and the syrup will keep like any other canned fruit until it is used.

Children should be encouraged to take a sufficient quantity of fluid, as the want of it is very apt to cause constipation. It is needless to say they should never touch alcohol in any form unless it is prescribed by a physician or is used in an emergency.

Elizabeth Robinson Scovil *The Care of Children*

CHAPTER V

THE FOOD OF SCHOOL CHILDREN

It has been well said that "children in school are more or less like animals in captivity." They are existing under artificial conditions of cramped position, and forced stillness of body and stimulation of mind, and too often deprived by bad ventilation of a fair share of the oxygen that is necessary to maintain vitality.

Under these circumstances their diet becomes a matter of increased importance.

When children live much in the open air, and are permitted to run about and exercise their bodies at their own free will, their appetites may safely be trusted to demand the food that is required for their support.

If we if we deprive them of these advantages we must see, at least, that they have nourishing, easily assimilated food, prepared in such a palatable manner that they will be induced to eat it.

THE PURPOSE OF FOOD

Food serves two great purposes:
- to build up flesh and bones, nerves, and blood.
- to furnish heat and power to the body.

The first end is accomplished by protein, a substance found abundantly in lean meat, fish, eggs, milk, cheese, and in some vegetables and meals, as peas, beans, oatmeal, wheat flour, rye and corn meal.

Heat and energy are furnished partly by fats, as cream, oil, butter, and the fat of meat; and partly by starch, contained in potatoes, many of the cereals, rice, tapioca, etc., and by sugar.

Children, from their ceaseless activity, require a large amount, proportionately, of the latter class of food.

Fortunately, many articles of diet contain both classes of food materials, as wheat bread, Indian meal, oatmeal, peas, beans, etc.

It is not the most expensive food that is most nourishing, and the mother of moderate means may give her child all the substances necessary to develop his body as well as the millionaire. It only requires a little knowledge, care and thought to do so.

Breakfast

It is very important that school children should lay a good foundation for the day's work in a substantial breakfast. This does not necessarily include meat. Indeed, hot meat once a day is enough for children. Protein can be given them in a less concentrated form.

The place of meat may be well supplied by fish. Many kinds are rich and nutritive properties. Fresh and salt cod fish, mackerel, blue fish, haddock, herring, shad, etc., are all useful.

In a seaport town fish can be obtained in perfection; farther inland its freshness is sometimes doubtful and then it should of course be rejected. This objection does not apply to salt or pickled fish.

The meal should begin with the porridge of some cereal and milk followed by fish or bacon with bread or toast and butter, not hot rolls, and conclude with fruit if it is obtainable.

Fruit consists principally of agreeable flavored water, but as this is very necessary in the animal economy its value must not be underrated.

The beverage should be cocoa, chocolate, hot or cold milk, diluted with water if preferred.

Luncheon

Children's luncheons require special thought. They should furnish about one fourth of the food material consumed during the day and, being eaten at a time when the body is a little tired, should be particularly appetizing.

Hot soup is desirable, but the practical difficulties in the way of providing a hot lunch are almost insurmountable.

When parents recognize the importance of insisting that the bodies as well as the minds of their children shall be developed at school, food will be provided there as one of the means to the end. Until then the mother must furnish the lunch basket.

The basis of the meal, for so it should be considered, and not merely as an unimportant morsel to be snatched by the way, must be sandwiches.

These can be made of thin bread and butter, brown or white, spread with minced or finely cut meat, sliced cheese, boiled or scrambled egg, preserved fruit, delicately shredded fish, sprinkled with salt, and sometimes a favored vegetable, as celery or lettuce.

Fresh fruit should be given whenever possible. A jelly tumbler with a tin top will hold a baked apple, stewed pear, prunes or any similar dainty.

Elizabeth Robinson Scovil *The Care of Children*

A suitable bottle should contain a glass of sterilized milk, or cocoa. A few crackers, or plain cookies, can be added; the aim being to have as much variety as possible.

The sandwiches should be wrapped in a napkin (those made from an old tablecloth do very well), and everything be as neat as possible. Nothing is small in the education of a child, and care in these trifling details will be well repaid by the taste for the refinements of life that it helps to cultivate.

Dinner

A plate of hot soup should usher in the dinner. In every household where this save-all is unknown scraps are wasted every day that would be sufficient to furnish a bountiful supply for the whole family. Nothing comes amiss to the soup pot; bread, cold vegetables, even fish, can be utilized, and their presence be unrecognized in the combination of flavors that renders the dish so acceptable.

The soup should be followed by meat roasted, boiled, stewed, or broiled; never fried, if it is possible to avoid it.

Meat may be recooked in various simple ways, as minced and baked with alternate layers of tomato, or cut thin, warmed in gravy and served on toast, or cut in slices, covered with gravy and baked in a deep pan with a thick covering of mashed potato. A well-made gravy is never greasy. Rich gravies and highly seasoned dishes, as curries, should be avoided for children.

With the meat there should be potatoes and one other vegetable; it matters little what so long as it is well cooked, neither over nor under done. Cabbage and turnips are rendered dark and strong smelling by too long cooking. Cabbage may be made almost as delicate as cauliflower by removing it from the fire as soon as it is tender. Changing the water once they're in the boiling prevents the disagreeable, characteristic odor during overcooking.

The meal may be concluded by a simple pudding, fruit, or ice cream. Pastry should be given very sparingly, but a perfectly healthy child may eat it occasionally with impunity, if it is good. Water is the only beverage that should be permitted at dinner.

Supper

There are two considerations that must be taken into account in preparing this repast. It is the last meal of the day and the child's digestion must not be overtaxed, or his sleep will be restless and uncomfortable. It is the last food he will have for twelve hours or more, and therefore must not be too slender in quantity or light in quality. Meat had better be avoided, particularly if it has been given at luncheon as well as at dinner. Eggs prepared in various ways are suitable, the cereals, if they are relished, bread and butter, milk toast, blanc mange, or custard, and fruit, fresh or stewed, preserves, honey or syrup.

Milk, hot or cold, and water are still the only liquids permissible.

AT BEDTIME

If a child plays hard and does not go to bed for two hours or more after supper, he may be hungry before he goes to sleep. In this case, it is wise to give a cracker and a glass of milk if they are desired.

Sometimes, alas, under our pernicious system of education, which obliges lessons to be learned at home, he, or more probably she, may be exhausted by an hour of study in the evening, and the tired brain will not easily quiet down to sleep. If this outrage on nature cannot be stopped, the evil effect may be a little modified by a glass of warm milk, which, setting the digestive organs in action, will draw away the blood from an over stimulated brain and render sleep possible.

CHAPTER VI

DIET IN ILLNESS

Food plays a very important part in the treatment of disease, even more important than medicine. In serious cases it will be prescribed by the doctor in attendance, but there are many in which it is well for the mother to know what diet is most suitable for the time being. In slight ailments a change of food is sometimes all that is needed to effect a cure.

Food in Constipation

This is one of the most frequent ills of childhood and one which can often be corrected by diet alone.

It is frequently caused by an insufficiency of water; not enough fluid is taken to flush the intestinal canal and help to carry off the waste matter. In these cases the child should have a glass of water early in the morning and several times during the day.

It can be flavored with fruit syrup, or a little sugar added, if it is not readily taken alone. The water may be either hot or cold.

Eggs, cheese and milk should be avoided for a time. These articles are thoroughly digested and absorbed by the system, leaving very little waste matter to be disposed of. This scanty remainder does not stimulate the intestines to action.

Vegetables and cereals leave more residue behind them and so give a greater bulk for the intestines to act upon.

Brown bread, oatmeal bread, or Graham bread, with butter and molasses, or syrup, oatmeal, or Indian meal porridge, stewed prunes, baked or stewed apples, any kind of fresh or stewed fruit, cream, soup, fresh meat, tomatoes and other vegetables may all be used to advantage.

A fig soaked overnight in a little water and given at breakfast before other food is an effectual remedy, the seeds acting as a stimulant.

If a baby is constipated, try half a teaspoonful of beef juice in its food twice a day, increasing the quantity to half a tablespoon if necessary.

Diarrhea

When a baby has diarrhea, look to the food; it is almost certainly in fault. Suspect the cleanliness of the nursing bottle, or the purity of the milk. Wash the one with redoubled care, sterilize the other, and boil any water used. If neither is guilty there may be some defect in the constituents of the food. Omit the cream for a day and increase the lime water.

If this is an ineffectual, stop giving the milk for a day and substitute rice water.

Should the symptoms still continue, do not waste more time; send for the doctor. With older children diarrhea often means that the digestive organs have been overtaxed with improper food or too great a quantity of it at once, and are trying to get rid of the offending substance. Except during the prevalence of cholera, when it should be attended to immediately, it may safely go unchecked for one day.

The diet should be light and unstimulating. Boiled milk may be given, grated flour ball, rice, tapioca, arrowroot, or sago, biscuit or crackers instead of bread, corn starch, barley gruel, junket, and, as the patient improves, boiled or baked custard.

Water should be drunk sparingly; ice may be taken to quench the thirst.

Avoid all the articles of food recommended for constipation.

ARROWROOT

This is a useful food in diarrhea, although, as it contains a large amount of starch, it is not suitable for very young babies.

To make it, mix a dessertspoonful of arrowroot to a smooth paste with cold water. Pour boiling water on it from the kettle, stirring until it thickens,. The water must be boiling hard or it will remain liquid. Add a little salt and sugar if desired.

If a spoon is left in it the thick gruel will become thin again.

INDIGESTION

Indigestion in babies is usually caused by improper food, as when starchy and farinaceous substances are used, which the baby cannot digest because it has no saliva to act upon them. Milk properly prepared with cream and lime water, or peptonized and given in the exact quantity required by the special baby in question, will usually effect a cure.

In older children the food must still bear the blame if there is indigestion.

Some bad habits contribute to it. One of the worst of these is eating too fast, which works harm in two ways. The food stays in the mouth so short a time the saliva does not have a chance to convert the starch into sugar; It is carried into the stomach, which nature has not fitted to deal with it in this condition, and there sets

Elizabeth Robinson Scovil *The Care of Children*

up an irritation and causes discomfort, as misplaced matter always does. When the food is hurried through the mouth it cannot be properly masticated, or ground by the teeth, and hard masses are sent to the stomach which it is beyond the power of that organ to separate. It grumbles at having to do work that does not belong to it, and we resent the just remonstrance and call it pain and indigestion.

Sometimes, of course, disease unfits the stomach to do its work, but this is not often the case, at least in the beginning, with children.

Those who suffer from indigestion should eat a small quantity at a time and have meals more frequently than those in health.

Toast soaked in beef or mutton juice, rare roast beef or mutton finely minced, the white meat of chicken, fresh fish that can be boiled, like cod fish or haddock, oysters, stale bread, plain puddings, rice, tapioca and oatmeal porridge with milk may be tried.

Avoid giving too great a variety at one time. One or two viands are enough at once.

Fat meat, cheese, fresh bread, much butter or cream, pastry, nuts, and any meat that has been warmed over, should not be given. Potato should be mashed. When it is certain that any article of food disagrees with the child its use should be forbidden. Only experience can decide which these are.

There should be as little discussion about the food as possible before the child.

Food in Rickets

As ricketts is a disease resulting chiefly from an improper diet, the food is a matter of prime importance. The first symptoms, which are described elsewhere, usually appear when a child is about six months old.

If the baby is being nursed he should be weaned, as the mother's milk is not nourishing him properly, or the food from the breast should be supplemented by alternate meals of malted milk, cream food, or barley food, or albumenized milk. A teaspoonful of beef juice should be given three times a day.

Salt should never be forgotten in the food.

The development of the bones being interfered with, material should be supplied to build them up and strengthen them. They are largely composed of earthy salts, or phosphates, which are contained abundantly in vegetables and grains, particularly in wheat, Indian corn, peas and potatoes.

Babies between six months and one year old may have bread, finely crumbled, and milk. Indian meal gruel, made with milk, cream and milk in abundance, diluted with lime water if necessary.

After a year old the child may have well-cooked pea soup, whitefish, if it can be obtained fresh, particularly haddock, boiled and shredded, baked potato, corn meal, cracked wheat, oatmeal porridge, bread and butter, a plentiful supply of the latter, as fat is desirable, milk and cream.

Dr. Emmet advises fat pork as a substitute for cod liver oil, which is often prescribed in these cases. Take a thick piece, free from lean, soak for thirty-six hours, changing the water frequently to get rid of the salt. Boil slowly, changing the water several times for eight hours. When cold it may be cut very thin and used in sandwiches, between thin slices of bread, sprinkled with salt; or rubbed to a paste and spread on the bread.

Well-made soup is suitable, particularly pea or potato soup, good broth of any kind, and cheese as soon as the child can digest it.

Fat bacon toasted over the coals may be used in any fresh meat cooked rare and finely minced before being given to the child.

DIET IN COLDS

When a child is chilly, fretful and feverish, has some coryza, or discharge from the nose, and perhaps oppression on the chest, his diet should be carefully regulated. It is an old saying, evolved from the experience of our ancestors, "If you feed a cold you will have to starve a fever".

When there is a disinclination for food the stomach should have complete rest for a few hours. Young mothers may remember for their comfort that starvation is a very slow process and that a well-fed child may go without food for a day without suffering from the fast, if water is given as required.

When the appetite is languid in the child who has hitherto eaten well, nature says decidedly "No more food at present, thank you. The digestive organs want the holiday." And we had better heed her indications. As a desire to eat returns, bread and milk, farina or hominy gruel, soup, or oyster broth, can be given.

When there is great thirst, flaxseed tea, or barley water, either flavored with lemon, are grateful. Rice water with a little currant or raspberry jelly stirred in it may be more acceptable than plain water.

Milk and water will sometimes be taken when milk alone would be rejected.

DIET IN ECZEMA

There are various afflictions of the skin, as roseola or heat rash, urticaria, known also as nettle rash or hives, and different forms of erythema, or heat spots, which often alarm mothers. The skin of children is delicate and very sensitive, sympathizing with any disturbance of the system, particularly of the digestion. The diet, therefore, is the subject of importance in these cases, as very often some defect in it has produced the disorder.

Meat should be discontinued until the affliction has disappeared, sugar, or anything sweet, being given sparingly, and oatmeal should not be used in any form.

Milk should be chiefly relied upon; boiled rice, gelatin, blanc mange, an egg occasionally and bread, or crackers, being used to supplement it.

FOOD IN FEVER

It may be considered an invariable rule that if a child's temperature is 101°F, taken with the clinical thermometer which comes for the purpose, he should have only liquids until it falls to normal again, around 98.5°F.

Beef tea is a stimulant rather than a food, and being laxative in its effect is not used when diarrhea is present.

Milk fulfills every purpose and should be given in suitable quantities, according to the age of the child, every two hours. It may be diluted with lime water, Vichy, Apollinaris water, or seltzer water, peptonized or sterilized, if necessary.

If stimulant is ordered, it can be given in it, though not if the taste is disliked, as this would disgust the child with his principal means of support.

It can be flavored with a few drops of vanilla, rose water, essence of lemon, or cocoa added to it; given iced or heated.

The yolk, or the white, of an egg in proportion of one to each cup of milk, can be shaken with it, and by varying it in these different ways it will be better borne.

Koumiss — This preparation of milk can sometimes be retained when in other forms it disagrees with the child.

It can be bought of the druggist; but is more cheaply made at home and with care success is easy.

Dissolve the third of a yeast cake in a little warm water. Stir it into one quart of milk, as warm as when it comes from the cow. Add one tablespoonful of sugar. Pour the mixture into large beer bottles, filling them about three-quarters full, and stand them in a warm place, about 68°F, for twelve hours, to rise like bread. If it is too hot the milk will curdle, instead of rising into a soft, foamy mass. The process of fermentation has been carried too far and the preparation is unfit for use.

If not put into bottles with patented stoppers it must be kept tightly corked. In any case it must be kept on ice or in a very cool place, as the low temperature checks further fermentation. It must be opened carefully, as it flies. Koumiss resembles buttermilk in taste and this also is sometimes given when milk, containing the cream or fat, cannot be borne.

Matzoon is similar in its nature and can also be procured from a druggist.

When the little patient begins to long for solid food, but cannot have it, the milk or beef juice can be stiffened with gelatin, which immediately re-dissolves in the stomach, being a solid only in the mouth.

Beef juice is more nutritious than beef tea.

Food in Tuberculosis

Children who have a tendency, inherited or otherwise, to consumption require special care in dieting.

The object is to build up the tissues, particularly those of the lungs, and render them unsuitable soil for the growth of the germ by which the disease is conveyed.

Fat is a very important element in their food, and as much must be given as can be digested. Cream, butter, bacon and eggs, especially the yolk, are some of the forms in which it can usually be easily taken. Bread is sometimes liked soaked in bacon fat, or spread with marrow which has been broiled on the bone. Older children may have lettuce with mayonnaise dressing, and a taste for salad oil should be cultivated. Some children will eat it on spinach or other green vegetables.

Cocoa and chocolate contain fat and are useful as the beverage. Plenty of milk should be given, fresh meat, and the cereals, as oatmeal, hominy, cracked wheat, farina, Indian meal, etc., may be made into porridge and eaten with cream.

The child should not be allowed to eat when tired, which is another way of saying that no violent exercise, or over-exertion, should be permitted near the mealtime.

Too great a variety of foods should not be given at once. Three or four articles are sufficient.

If there is a distaste for solid food, more milk, uncooked eggs, white or yolk, preferably the latter, can be given, and beef or mutton broth, or any good vegetable soup, particularly pea or bean soup.

Artificial goat's milk is made by adding two tablespoonfuls of beef suet, minced fine, to one pint of milk. This is brought to the boil and allowed to simmer for a short time, stirring constantly. If too much fat floats on the top, a little may be skimmed off. Salt is added, or a little celery salt, if the taste is light, and the milk drunk when hot.

CLOTHING
CHAPTER VII

THE BABY'S WARDROBE

The young mother is often puzzled to know exactly what clothes will be needed by the newcomer and how they can best be provided.

If a woman can sew neatly, has plenty of time, a little ingenuity, and is well enough to work with ease, it is a pleasure to her to make the dainty little garments herself. If the conditions are not favorable, it is better to buy the outfit ready made than to employ a seamstress, as this makes it much more expensive.

The looser a baby's garments are the more comfortable they will be. Modern patterns entirely dispensed with the bands in which the tender body used to be tightly pinned, and the gain to the baby, in comfort is at least if nothing more, is very great.

It is sometimes difficult for an inexperienced person to procure the right patterns. One for a plain slip, another for a Mother Hubbard dressed with a yoke, and, if needed, a pattern for the little shirt, can easily be obtained from any large house dealing with cut paper patterns. With these the whole outfit can be successfully fashioned.

If materials cannot readily be procured in a small town or village, samples will be sent on application to any dry goods store in a city, and from these the choice can be made as easily and almost says satisfactorily as if seated at the counter.

The label on the pattern states the quantity of the material required. There is one drawback to these models, the skirts are too long. Thirty inches from the neck to hem is amply long for the outside dress, and the undergarments may be two to three inches shorter period allowance must be made for this in estimating the amount of material that will be needed.

The wardrobe should consist of:

3 Bands,	48 Napkins,
2 wrappers,	Cloak,
4 skirts,	6 Night Slips,
Socks,	Hood,
6 Petticoats,	8 Dresses.
Blankets,	

This supply will be ample if the washing is done at home. If it has to be sent to a laundry, it is better to add a dozen napkins, two night slips, four Dresses, and two shirts.

BANDS

These are only required for a week or two to keep the dressing in place. It is a great mistake to think that the abdominal walls must be held immovable by a tight bandage. Nature has constructed them to support themselves. The band, as usually applied, increases the danger of rupture by pressing down the contents of the abdomen against the weak points, and so bringing about the very accident it was meant to guard against.

As they are to be used so short a time, three strips of soft flannel, torn off and not finished in any way, are all that is necessary. The knitted bands preferred by some mothers are difficult to keep in place, being apt to work up under the arms in an uncomfortable ridge.

SHIRTS

Many of the reformed systems of baby clothes dispense with the shirt, substituting for it a flannel slip with sleeves. The disadvantage is that if the long garment gets wet the baby must be undressed and have it removed. The short shirt is well out of harm's way.

Those of ribbed cashmere, high neck, long sleeves and opening all the way down the front, are the best, even for the summer baby. They cost from forty-five to seventy-five cents each, and better quality wear very well. Silk and wool ones can be purchased, but of course they're more expensive, and have no special advantage except added daintiness.

In putting on a shirt, it is wise to fasten it behind, as then the sleeves of all garments can be fitted into one another and put on as one. Fasten it with a safety pin to the napkin in front to help keep it from slipping up.

The shirts can be made by the pattern from cotton and wool or silk and wool flannel, the seams being laid flat and each side neatly cat stitched in place. They can be bound with silk flannel binding, which washes better than ribbon.

Flannel containing cotton or silk shrinks less than that of all wool and so is preferable for an infant's garments. The cotton and wool costs about thirty-five cents a yard, silk and wool from sixty-five cents to a dollar. At the latter price it is beautifully fine and pretty enough for a cloak or outside other outside garment.

Shirts should be worn at night as well as in the day, one being kept for each service, unless a flannel night dress is used.

Petticoats

These are replaced in the modern outfit by sleeveless flannel slips, opening in the back, made with large arm holes, which are buttonholed with soft silk, cat stitched or bound. In cutting them by a slip pattern make the armholes larger and the neck lower than is indicated, finishing the ladder to match the armholes. The bottom should be finished with a plain two-inch hem.

In another model the front and back are cut alike, the opening being on the shoulders. The shoulder seams are cut deeper to allow for lapping and fastened with tiny buttons and button holes. If the slip has to be removed during the day, the hands can be passed under the loose dress, the buttons undone and the garment slipped off without removing the dress.

If it is desired, one or two white slips can be made of Lonsdale cambric to wear on state occasions, as the dress looks rather prettier over them. They are not needed ordinarily.

Napkins

The material that is variously known as Canton flannel, cotton flannel and swansdown, is a good one for napkins. It is soft and absorbent. The thinner quality, costing about seven-cents a yard, is the best to use for this purpose. Squares are made the width of the material, about twenty-five inches, and hemmed on two sides. These can be folded twice at first. For a young baby napkins may be made of soft linen, as an old tablecloth. These should be thirty-five inches long by seventeen inches wide, being doubled to make the square before they are folded.

Cotton and linen diaper, or birdseye, as it is also called, are used; the latter is cold and does not absorb the moisture well.

Stockinet napkins can be procured for this purpose at some of the larger dry goods stores. They are good, but more expensive than those made of the other fabrics that have been mentioned. They must not be confounded with stockinette diapers, which have a coating of rubber on one side.

India rubber prevents the moisture from evaporating and causes the wet cloth to act like a poultice to the others to the tender skin. Waterproof napkins may save the baby's clothing from being damp, but they also are so injurious they should not be tolerated by the careful mother.

A square of thick flannel is an additional protection and does no harm. One will be found very useful at night.

Pads

A piece of soft old a piece of soft old cotton or linen, folded to a square, may be placed inside the napkin. If it is soiled It can be rolled up and burned, thus saving much disagreeable washing. If only wet, it can be sent to the laundry.

Napkins should not be used a second time without being washed. There is a solid deposit, invisible to the naked eye, which remains after the moisture has dried, and is apt to chafe and irritate the skin.

Night Slips

These are best made perfectly plain, without a yoke, the fullness at the neck being gathered into a band. This may be edged with soft lace if desired and a few tucks added above the hem at the bottom.

Lonsdale cambric, about sixteen cent a yard, is a good material to use for them. The baby will need no other dress during the first month, the one worn in the day being changed for another at night if necessary. As the flannel slip is worn also, nothing warmer is needed.

Dresses

The absurd fashion of encumbering a little baby with long skirts is happily becoming a thing of the past. The weight was a serious matter to the delicate child and an unnecessary burden to a strong one. Thirty inches from neck to hem is amply long and it is no disadvantage to have them an inch or two shorter, if the underslips are made to correspond.

Nainsook muslin costing about fifty to seventy-five cents a yard is a very pretty material for them. Victoria lawn can be used and fine Lonsdale cambric is less expensive. There is a muslin with a fine cord and hair line, that makes serviceable garments, but checks and figures should be avoided.

The dresses should be made with yokes, or full in front and back, with the fullness laid in fine tucks to the waistline.

The first requisite for a baby's dress is to be loose, so as to be easily slipped on and off.

They may be trimmed with narrow lace or Hamburg edging. Deeper embroidery is not considered in good taste. A tiny vine embroidered by hand is admissible. Hemp stitching is an appropriate decoration. Feather stitching is an appropriate decoration. Feather stitching between clusters of tucks always looks well. A machine-made feather stitching can be purchased, which saves many stitches. It can be put on each side of narrow Hamburg intersection insertion, or between clusters of tucts.

Elizabeth Robinson Scovil *The Care of Children*

Yokes can be bought ready made and the skirts added. This is an easy way to make dresses, as the yokes are troublesome except to an expert needlewoman.

If a specially handsome dress is required, it is best to get it ready for use.

WRAPPERS

There is nothing prettier in all the baby's outfit than the dainty little wrappers. They are useful to slip on early in the morning, or to put over the dress when the room is cooler than usual.

A cut paper pattern is easily obtained by writing to any firm that deals in patterns.

They may be made with the yolk and the skirt pulled on, of course opening in front, or cut wide enough to tuck the front, or lay it in three plaits on each side with a box plait in the back.

Silk and wool flannel, cashmere, opera flannel, Scotch flannel, outing cloth and Shaker flannel are all suitable materials, the latter two being very inexpensive.

They may be feather stitched, embroidered in a delicate pattern, or trimmed with lace, and tied with ribbon. There is room for the exercise of much taste and ingenuity in color and decoration.

SOCKS

There are strong arguments for and against covering the feet of little babies with socks. They are apt to become wet and so uncomfortable. But they can be changed when the napkin is and sometimes escape altogether.

It is urged that if the baby is active and they are kicked off, unless tied too tightly for the good of the tiny foot. There is a happy medium of tightness by which they can be made tolerably secure and yet not impede the circulation. It is important that the feet should be kept warm and, although this may be partially done by pinning together the edges of the flannel slip, the socks are a great additional protection.

Anyone who can knit or crochet can make them out of white zephyr, or stouter ones from single Germantown wool, ornamenting them if desired with pink, blue, pale yellow, or crimson trimmings. Those who are not skilled in fancy work can procure a pattern and cut them from stockinette or half-worn stocking-legs, feather-stitching the seams with embroidery silk and any color desired.

The best parts of a discarded undershirt may be utilized for the purpose, if it is soft and comparably thick.

Too many pair cannot be provided; at least a dozen are needed, for holes develop with marvelous rapidity when the little feet are constantly in motion.

Blankets

Kind friends are almost sure to provide one or two pretty, dainty ones of silk and wool, or fine all wool flannel, hem stitched or embroidered with flowers and leaves in satin stitch. These are delightful to possess for state occasions but will not stand the wear and tear of everyday use.

For this there is nothing better than blankets knitted from single Germantown wool. They should be, when finished, three-quarters of a yard wide and a yard long.

They are knitted on rubber or bone needles quarter of an inch in diameter. Set up 123 stitches and knit backwards and forwards and plain knitting, or any fancy stitch preferred, until the desired length is attained. Stripes of pink, blue, or yellow are pretty knitted near the ends, but soon lose their color in washing. Rows of narrow ribbon can be run in instead and taken out when the blanket is soiled.

Those who prefer crocheting to knitting can use it.

Plain blankets can be made of cotton and wool flannel with a two-inch hem feather stitched with washing silk.

Blankets are only useful for the first month or two, while the baby is content to keep comparatively still.

Little jackets, which looks so pretty and dainty when they are first made, soon lose their freshness. They are easily soiled and difficult to put on and take off. When a cashmere shirt and flannel slip are used they are not needed for warmth.

Cloaks

There is a great diversity of opinion as to when a baby should first go out of doors. Much, of course, depends upon the season of the year. What would be perfectly safe proceeding at mid-summer would be of great risk in winter. If the house is in good sanitary condition and the room used as a nursery is well ventilated, there is no necessity for the baby being carried into the open air until it is six weeks or two months old. Nor need it be taken out at all in very cold weather.

It is well to provide the cloak and the hood beforehand, as the mother has plenty of cares to occupy her time and attention with the arrival of the baby.

Nothing is as pretty as white for the first cloak. It may be made of cream cashmere or any soft all wool material, and trimmed with a fringe of ribbon loops, or stripes of ribbon, about four inches in length, laid on the skirt and cape from the edge upward, with feather stitching done in embroidery silk between. In winter it may be trimmed with narrow bands of white fur.

The cloak should be lined with Canton flannel when warmth is necessary, and with cream-colored cambric or percale in summer. Cloaks can be purchased ready made for little more than it costs to buy the material, and, unless the mother is skillful needlewoman, it is the wisest to do this.

Hoods

Dainty little hoods may be bought at comparatively small expense. They are made of cashmere to match the cloak, or of soft cream or white silk, or of embroidered muslin with a thin silk lining for the summer baby.

All have full frills of lace around the face and are tied with ribbon.

If it is desired to make the hood at home, a paper pattern can easily be obtained. The saving is not very great, and making it is a difficult task to accomplish neatly.

Mittens

The winter baby must have its hands covered when it goes out, and it is a wise precaution whenever the weather is cool. The dainty mittens of white, pink, or blue are as fascinating as the socks. They are easily made by a skillful knitter and cost about twenty-five cents a pair when purchased.

CHAPTER VIII

SHORT CLOTHES

When a strong, active baby is between four and five months old, it is time to put it in short clothes. Even moderately long shirts impede its motion to some extent and should be discarded.

SHIRTS

The cashmere shirt is still worn, over that a flannel slip, with long sleeves in winter and short ones in the summer. In very hot weather a cotton one may be substituted. These slips are cut princess shape, reaching nearly to the ankles, and are sloped a in a little at the waist.

If desired, a band can be stitched on at the waistline, buttons sewn on it and a cambric petticoat buttoned on.

Napkins must be retained for some time to come. When they are left off little drawers may replace them, but this cannot be until the baby has learned good habits.

WAISTS

Some mothers prefer a waist buttoning behind, with buttons on the lower edge to which the skirt and drawers can be attached. These should be made double, of cotton, quite loose and not corded or stiffened in any way. In this case a flannel petticoat is used instead of the slip and the waist may be of flannel for the winter baby.

Sometimes, until the child leaves off napkins and requires the waist to support drawers, two flannel slips are used, one with sleeves, and the other without, and the shirt is dispensed with.

DRESSES

Many mothers think it is most economical to shorten the long dresses. If they are likely to be needed again it is best to lay them aside for future use and make new ones, perhaps of rather stouter material, at least for everyday wear. These should come to the ankles, just showing the feet.

White is still the prettiest color and at first the most suitable. When washing is an item to be considered, others may be substituted.

For the summer baby, beside Lonsdale muslin, lawn, nainsook or any pretty muslin in stripe or small check; cottons, cambrics, percales, etc., and delicate colors with fine lines, dots or tiny figures, can be used.

The winter baby looks well in dresses of Shaker flannel, Scotch flannel, in narrow stripes, plain cashmere of any tint preferred, or other soft all wool material, plain or in small pattern. Plaids or any striking effects should not be tolerated in a baby's dresses.

White cashmere makes a useful best dress, as it looks well if carefully washed, and can be dyed when its freshness is gone beyond recall. Any fabric that will not wash is unsuited for a baby's dress.

The short dresses look well made with square or pointed yolks, and little skirts being gathered on them. For older babies these yokes are sometimes trimmed with a deep thrill extending over the shoulders, giving something to the effect of a guimpe.

The bottom of the skirt may have a cluster of narrow tucks above a wide hem.

CREEPING SKIRTS

When a baby begins to creep it is impossible to keep the dress tidy and clean without some protection. This is best afforded by a creeping skirt. Dark cotton or gingham is a suitable material to use, as it must be capable of being washed and not too heavy. It is made of two widths of cotton, perfectly straight, like a bag, only open at both ends, with the string case at each end. Broad elastics are run in these and the skirt put on over the dress, the other end being brought up round the waist under the petticoats, enclosing them like a bag. It can be slipped off in a moment, leaving the dress comparatively fresh.

BIBS

When teething begins there is usually an extra secretion of saliva and it's difficult to keep the front of the dress dry. Bibs may be made of linen diaper lined with cotton flannel shrunk before using. They can be made of fine Lonsdale cambric or nainsook muslin,, with the thin layer of wadding between it and the cotton lining and quilted in diamonds, or a pattern, either on the sewing machine or by hand. They cost much less than to buy.

When there is so much moisture that the bid quickly becomes soaked with it, making the dress damp, it is a good plan to have a bib, cut the same shape, of white India rubber cloth to wear beneath it. The edges can be bound with silk binding if desired.

This material makes a convenient feeding bib for older children, as it can be wiped with a damp cloth and does not require washing. White table oil cloth may be used for the same purpose and is less expensive.

CLOAKS

The long white cloak is laid aside with the long dresses, and, although white is still pretty and suitable, colors may be used.

Jersey, or eiderdown flannel is an excellent material for winter, being soft and warm. It can be lined with Canton flannel, matching it in color.

White eiderdown is very pretty, trimmed with bands of beaver, either the real fur or the imitation plush, which closely resembles it. Red looks well with a narrow edging of black astrakhan, and blue with white angora fringe, or the curled gray astrakhan. The silky angora fringe can be obtained in different shades of steel and gray to match flannels of the same colors.

For summer, any thick white washing material that is desired may be used; new ones appear every year; and it can be trimmed with narrow braid, edged with embroidery, or simply with rows of machine stitching.

The fabrics mentioned for wrappers make excellent cloaks for a cool day.

BONNETS

These can be obtained in so many quaint and pretty shapes that the mother need never be at a loss for covering for the baby's head. It must be soft; nothing looks more forlorn than a stiff hat, straw or felt, on a very young child.

Dainty hoods may be made of the same material as the cloak and trimmed to match it, or they may be of silk, velvet, cashmere, or muslin, according to the season. There is ample opportunity for the exercise of individual tastes.

STOCKINGS

These should be long enough to cover the knees, and carefully chosen in regard to the size of the feet, that the toes may not be cramped. There is no reason why the foot should not be as symmetrical as the hand, the toes are little distorted as the fingers. It is only undue pressure that forces them out of shape, and corns are the effort that nature makes to protect the tender tissue, which never was meant to undergo such squeezing. Their foundation is too often laid in childhood.

The stockings may be of any color that is preferred. Black ones are much worn and look well with any shoes. They may be fastened to a button on the waist, or slip, with an elastic band, care being taken that it is not too tight.

SHOES

These may be made at home of chamois, felt and soft kid, shaped like a moccasin. They do not wear very well, but, as shoes are an expensive item in the baby's wardrobe, they may repay the trouble of making.

Elizabeth Robinson Scovil *The Care of Children*

When a baby begins to use the feet for standing and prepares to make an attempt to walk, something firmer is needed that will give more support to the foot. It is then that the mother's trials in the matter of foot-gear commence.

Diligent search must be made for a shoe that is broad enough in the sole not to cramp the foot and that makes a faint attempt to conform to the natural shape of it by, at least, having the sole flat and not rounded on the bottom. This peculiarity prevents the weight from being thrown upon the toes, where a part of it belongs, and brings it on the heel, the toes being scarcely able to touch the ground. The inside line of the sole should be nearly straight, not to bend the joint of the great toe out of place.

It is a pity that sandals ever went out of fashion, but, as they are gone, we can only try to supply their place with shoes broad enough to give the toes free play. Much emphasis is often laid on having the shoe sufficiently long. While this is important, no excess in length, beyond the limit of comfort, will make up for deficiency in width.

CHAPTER IX

CLOTHING AFTER BABYHOOD

BOYS' FROCKS

There is usually no distinction made between the dress of boys and girls until after they are two years old.

It is a mistake to put boys into sailor suits too early; they do not look well in them before they are at least three years old. They are a saving of trouble, and, if the mother is overburdened, this is a great consideration.

Until then, there are many pretty ways in which the little dresses can be made, which do not look too girlish to be suitable for boys.

The simplest is a plain front with full back, the fullness held in place by two straps, coming from the side seams and crossing behind. This may have either a round collar or one cut in two squares in front and in behind and trimmed with braid or embroidery.

Another has the plaited kilt skirt and a blouse falling over it. The blouse may have jacket fronts, opening over a full vest, the fronts being rounded or square, as desired.

An effective pattern buttons diagonally from the neck to hem in front, the skirt being full behind and having the fullness laid in two box plaits, the joining with the waist being concealed by straps coming from the side seams and buttoning in the back.

A very pretty suit has a box plaited skirt and blouse with sailor collar, having long points in front that extend to the waistline.

In one of the prettiest the waist has three box plates in front and behind, the skirt being box plaited also, finished with a plain belt, buttoned in front, and a little round collar.

The front of the dress may hang straight, with three boxed plaits, the back being gathered on a plain waist with belt from the side seams, crossing behind.

BOYS' FIRST SUITS

When a boy grows too large for skirts, the next garment is a sailor suit, consisting of a blouse and knee breeches, or long trousers, as preferred.

The material may be navy blue or gray flannel, light-weight tweed, or soft woolen fabric, velveteen, serge, either blue or white, and linen duck, blue denim, or any stout cotton material, for summer.

Boys enjoy the freedom of trousers and are always charmed to assume them as a step towards the manliness they all aspire to.

The suits should be supplied with pockets and can usually be purchased almost as cheaply as they can be made. It is often possible to get an extra pair of trousers and sometimes pieces for patching are sold with them.

When the mother's inspiration fails her, she should send for a catalogue of children's fashions and glean ideas from that. The points to remember in dressing children are to have the clothing loose, the weight supported principally by the shoulders, and not to overload the dresses with trimming. Simplicity is not only the most sensible, but it is in the best taste.

LITTLE GIRLS' DRESSES

In little girls' dresses the belts of the boys are replaced by sashes, coming from the side seams and tied behind. The waists are shorter than in boys, and very often an overdress is made to wear over a guimpe, or yoke and sleeves, of another material.

Sometimes the fullness is simply shirred at the neck, or the skirt is gathered on a yoke, and there are two deep frills round the neck, the lower one extending over the shoulders.

The materials are much the same for both sexes, gingham, chambray, linen, or any pretty cotton goods, Navy blue, or fancy flannel, soft all wool fabric; and for little girls China or India silk, or light woolen materials, may be used.

Children should not be dressed in such a way as to oblige them to think of their clothes. The play dresses should be strong, not to tear easily, and washable, so that a visit to the laundry will restore their freshness. Close contact with mother earth is essential to the health and well-being of all young, growing things, and the thought of danger to clothes should never have to stand in the way of it with boys and girls.

UNDERCLOTHING

High necked undershirts, varying in weight from thick cashmere in winter to thinnest gauze in very hot weather, should be insisted on upon. They need not be long sleeved in summer. The chest must be protected, but the forearm is not a vital part. Drawers should be worn in cold weather, but are not essential for boys in warm. Some mothers preferred the union suits, shirts and drawers in one. Over the undergarment, boys, after they have put on knickerbockers, wear a cotton shirt, either white or of soft, twilled, colored material, and girls a waist.

It cannot be too earnestly impressed upon the mind of the mother that girls should never wear tight fitting waists, nor corsets. No woman ever acknowledged that her corsets were tight, but no matter how loose they are, they interfere with the proper development of the growing girl, render her figure less pliant and graceful, and destroy the easy carriage that is such a charm.

A comfortable waist with shoulder straps and buttons, on which the flannel petticoat, underskirt and drawers can be buttoned, does no harm and furnishes all the support that is necessary. If the muscles never have been weakened by the inaction that pressure maintains, they are abundantly able to support themselves and their owner too.

The dresses may be of any shape that is liked, provided there are no tight bands about the waist.

If mothers only realize how important it is that the delicate organs should have free play, utterly untrammeled by pressure from without, and knew the disastrous consequences that must follow any infringement of nature's laws, they would be the very first to insist upon a rigid adherence to sensible methods of dress.

Stockings

When economy is a necessity, a slight saving may be effected by purchasing stockings out of season, summer ones in the autumn and winter ones in the spring; they are often sold at a reduction to prevent the necessity of packing them away.

Black is, on the whole, the most satisfactory, although navy blue and dark brown look well for boys with suits of the same colors. Those purchased for boys should be stout, cotton or woolen, according to the time of year; ribbed ones fit the leg better than plain. Knee pads are a great protection when short trousers are worn. They are shaped to fit over the knee and are made of leather, or thick felt, being worn under the trousers.

Some mothers line the heels of the new stockings with the piece of Canton flannel, cut to fit, to prevent their wearing so quickly.

A pattern can be obtained for cutting over old stockings for a smaller foot. A part of the leg is utilized for the upper part of the foot and heel, a new sole being cut and sewed in.

Stocking supporters hold the stockings firmly in place.

Little girls may wear hose to match their dresses in color. Cotton or lisle thread in summer, cashmere or woolen in winter. It is of the utmost importance to keep the feet warm. It is well to remember, in purchasing stockings of an unusual shade, to buy cotton, or worsted, for the same with which to darn them.

It is more economical to get cotton by the ball and wool in skeins, rather than a small quantity on cards.

SHOES

All that has been said on the importance of not cramping the baby's feet applies with added force to those of the growing boy and girl, who are constantly using theirs.

The shoes should be comfortably long and wide, being careful that they fit well. Too much room is almost as bad as too little. The heels must be low and flat, that the weight of the body may not be thrown too far forward in walking.

High French heels should not be tolerated for little girls. No boy would endure them.

It is a mistake to have too heavy shoes. They tire the feet unnecessarily. The soles should be stout enough to protect from dampness. As the use of rubber overshoes is almost universal, they need not be so thick as to keep out water.

It is good economy, when it is possible, to have two pairs of shoes that can be worn alternatively. Have them kept well brushed and cleaned. In buying the patent dressing, try to procure one that contains glycerin, as this helps to prevent the leather from cracking. A little Vaseline, well rubbed in before an ordinary dressing is applied, serves the same purpose.

Bedroom slippers must not be forgotten, as running around in bare feet is a dangerous pastime.

They may be crocheted, or knitted, of Germantown wool and have lamb's wool shoe soles. But red or black felt ones cost very little more and are far more durable.

Pretty fancy leather ones can be purchased in red, blue or yellow, to match the wrapper.

Long rubber boots are very desirable for wet weather. Lamb's wool soles can be slipped in them, rendering a shoe unnecessary. No rubber foot covering should be worn for any length of time; as in sitting in school. There is no escape for the moisture caused by the perspiration, and the feet soon become damp. Rubber overshoes are especially necessary for girls, as wet feet are a distinct source of danger to them.

It is said that when shoes are wet they should be freed from mud as much as possible, well rubbed with kerosene oil and put where they will dry slowly; when partially dry, they should be rubbed with the oil again, and that this renders the leather soft and pliable.

APRONS

These useful garments have rather gone out of fashion at the present moment, but they are too convenient not to be restored to favor. High-necked, long-sleeved aprons of striped gingham, or blue and white cotton, are a great protection to the child at play, and when soiled can be easily replaced.

A pretty white one that can be slipped on at a moment's notice makes a plain dress presentable.

There are so many patterns for little girls, the mother has only to choose between them. White muslin, plain, checked, or striped, or lawn trimmed with narrow lace, embroidery, or ruffles of the same, always look well and come from the laundry almost as good as new.

Black silk aprons, high-neck and with long sleeves, are fancied for schoolgirls. They can be ornamented with feather stitching and black or color, and finish with rows of shirring or smocking around the neck. They served to protect the dress, particularly the sleeves, which are soon worn and soiled by rubbing on the desk.

WRAPPERS

These are useful for little children to be slipped on early in the morning, when they want to run around before being dressed. They can be made of Jersey or eiderdown flannel, for winter, or of Scotch flannel lined with cotton flannel. For summer, nothing is nicer than outing flannel, so-called, though it does not contain a threat of wool.

A girl always requires a wrapper, and it may be made of any of the pretty, soft materials used for her mother's. Boys usually despise them, except an illness, until they are grown up and begin to appreciate the luxuries of bath robe and lounging jacket.

NIGHTGOWNS

This is an important part of the children's wardrobe, as they pass more than one-third of their lives in bed, and does not always receive the attention it deserves.

In winter, for young children, they should be of white or gray flannel, made very long, extending at least half a yard below the feet. There may be a string case at the bottom, and the string, being loosely tied, converts to garment into a kind of bag, impossible to kick off and rendering exposure to cold and accident no longer to be feared. In the morning the superfluous length can be turned up and tied around the waist or under the arms.

Older children should wear night dresses of outing or Shaker flannel. If preferred, they may have an undershirt of the same weight as the one worn during the day, being sure that a different one is kept for the night, and always changed.

A good substitute is an over jacket of any light flannel; some children dislike the friction of any material thicker than cotton next to the skin.

Except in the warmest weather, a single cotton garment is not sufficient protection at night. Delicate, nervous children, especially, require additional clothing, or else the nervous energy, so precious to them, is expended in keeping the body warm, when proper covering would prevent the escape and waste of the heat already generated.

Outer Garments

A boy should be provided with two overcoats — a thick ulster for winter, and one of lighter weight for the intermediate seasons. A rubber coat is useful when there is prolonged exposure to rain, as in a long walk to school. No boy likes to play in one, particularly if those important personages, "the other boys", do not wear them. Its place may be filled by a thick reefer.

A girl needs a warm cloak for winter. If she lives in a cold climate, it should be supplemented by a jacket of chamois skin, lined with silk or alpaca, that it may slip on easily, and covered with flannel or any woolen material desired. If the cloak can be fur trimmed, so much the better; it should have a high collar to protect the back of the neck.

An ulster of long rubber cloth garment is indispensable for rainy days.

Girls should have one or two blazers or light jackets for cool days in summer, as well as the thinner cloth ones that are necessary for spring and autumn.

Hats

It is always puzzling to the young mother to know what headgear best benefits the dignity of the baby boy after he has outgrown the silk or cashmere hood in which he looked so sweet at first.

In summer he may have a linen sun hat for everyday wear, and a silk Tam o' Shanter or a soft cap with a hexagonal crown for best. These can be replaced in winter by a little velvet cap, trimmed with a fur band to match his coat.

When he is two years old, he may be advanced to a sailor hat of straw or felt, or wear one of the quaint shapes, as the three-cornered Continental, that change with each successive year.

Bonnets of silk, velvet or cashmere are still the prettiest for little girls, in cold weather. When it is warmer, they can be exchanged for the Normandy muslin caps with high, peaked crown, that are so becoming to the dear little faces. The linen sun hats will be found very useful for them, too, as they can be washed without difficulty.

Older children should be allowed some expression of their own choice in clothes, particularly in the matter of head covering. What seems a detail of perfect indifference to the mother may mean an agony of mortification to the sensitive boy or girl. In no case is it more necessary for us to be able to put ourselves in another's place than in dealing with the idiosyncrasies of children.

In selecting a hat for a girl, it is well to remember that it must be worn with several dresses and should not look out of place with any of them. To accomplish this, it must be quiet in tone and not too conspicuous in shape. Ribbon or velvet, with perhaps one or two ostrich tips, is a more appropriate trimming than artificial flowers.

The cruelty of wearing as an ornament the plumage of birds, which must be killed to obtain it, should be early impressed on the childish mind. The lesson will then never be forgotten.

Elizabeth Robinson Scovil *The Care of Children*

BEDS AND BEDDING
CHAPTER X

THE BED

As babies ought to spend the greater part of their time in sleep, the older children should pass at least ten hours out of the twenty-four in bed, the bed itself becomes a matter of importance.

Bassinets

Young mothers are always fascinated by the pretty, wicker bassinets, muslin trimmed and silk lined, that seem such cozy little nests for the tiny sleepers. They are very charming and, for those who can afford them, nothing can be prettier. This does not mean only afford the first cost, for that need not be excessive, but the tax on time and strength that renewing the dainty draperies involves. They begin to lose their freshness soon after the mother has assumed the sole charge of her new treasure, when every faculty is fully occupied with the necessary duties of each day. This slight additional demand seems like the proverbial last straw, and the mother is apt to wish she had chosen a couch with more durable decorations.

If one is desired, it can be bought ready for use at any large establishment where babies' outfits are sold; or it may be bought without covering and finished at home. A large oval clothes basket makes a good substitute.

The bassinet is lined with glazed cambric, pink, blue, or yellow as preferred, covered with dotted, figured, or plain muslin, either basted smoothly over it, or fulled on. Round the top of the basket there is a ruffle of silk or muslin to conceal the stitches that hold the lining in place. India, China or surah silk can be used instead of muslin. The basket sometimes has a canopy or a curved rod to support curtains, which are tied back with ribbon. A stout framework may be provided to hold it and draped to match the bassinet, or it may rest on a table, or two chairs. It has the advantage of being easily carried from room to room.

A pillow covered with a rubber case is the only bed required for the bassinet. A white pillowcase can be put on, or a little blanket folded over it. This, with a tiny pillow for the head, and a warm blanket or silk wadded comforter completes the outfit.

A large clothes basket, or large, low box, makes the safe and convenient receptacle for a baby when he is able to sit alone. It can be padded with pillows and the little occupant will stay in it contentedly for a long time with a few toys to amuse him.

CRIBS

A rattan or iron crib is the most sensible bed to purchase, for it can be used until the child has outgrown babyhood. Iron cribs painted white with brass finishings, look very well. They can be obtained fitted with rods for a canopy, which is always a pretty addition, besides protecting the head from draughts and the eyes from light. It can be made of rose-bud chintz, washing silk, India drapery, or any material that is liked.

The crib is usually fitted with the woven wire mattress, which makes the best foundation for any bed, and over this a soft hair mattress. A folded blanket should be laid on this. Next, a square of rubber cloth, or a pad, and over that the sheet. An upper sheet is not required, a soft blanket and dainty white quilt, not too heavy, supplying its place.

HAMMOCKS

A hammock makes a convenient bed for a baby where space is a consideration. Very elaborate ones are manufactured of silk and with heavy silken fringes, but the baby will sleep quite as comfortably in a small size, ordinary one.

A crib blanket forms the bed, with the rubber protector over it. A pillow is not needed. Two bands should be provided to tie around the hammock, rendering it impossible for the occupant to fall out of it. It can be suspended from two stout hooks screwed into the wall.

COMFORTERS

Babies need warmth without weight. For this reason, a down comforter makes a good covering in cool weather. It should frequently be hung out in the sun to air and, if the colors are delicate, may be protected by a slipcover of any washable material at night. A comforter of cheesecloth, wadded and tufted with zephyr of any color preferred is not expensive and can be changed when soiled.

Blankets — Small ones can be purchased of a proper size for cribs. It is best to cut the pair in two and finish the cut ends by binding them with narrow ribbon or buttonholing them with worsted matching the stripes and color.

When soiled they should be sent to a professional cleaner as they never look as well after home washing.

Elizabeth Robinson Scovil *The Care of Children*

Cream eiderdown flannel may be used instead of blankets. It is pretty bound with ribbon, but this is not very durable.

SHEETS

In hemming sheets, which the baby needs as he grows older, it is well to remember that if there is a broad hem at each end of the sheet can be reversed and wears more evenly than if the same end were always placed at the top. Cotton is much better than linen for this purpose.

Protectors — Rubber cloth costs about seventy-five cents a yard for a narrow width; if a cheaper material is required, white table oil cloth makes a good substitute. It is not as durable as the rubber cloth, but it's waterproof for a time.

Pads can be made of several thicknesses of newspaper, which answer the purpose very well, a fresh one being used when the old one becomes damp. They can be slipped into a cotton cover made for the purpose, which is easily washed.

PILLOWS

Pillows may be of down, feathers, or hair. A thin feather one is probably the best, giving softness without undue warmth.

A tiny square one looks pretty at first, and two large hem-stitched pocket handkerchiefs, men's size, make a dainty pillowcase.

Children should be taught to sleep with the head low as it helps to make them straight. One thin pillow is all that is necessary.

It is very important that a child should not be permitted to draw the bedclothes over the face. The exhalations from the body are breathed into the lungs instead of the fresh, pure air, laden with oxygen, with which the sleeping room ought to be filled.

BED CLOTHES FASTENERS

Patent bed-clothes fasteners can be purchased for a small sum, by which the upper coverings can be fastened to the bedstead in such a way that the child cannot throw them off.

Very large safety pins, such as are used for horse blankets, make a tolerable substitute. The clothes can be pinned to the mattress, but not drawn so tight as the interfere with the comfort of the sleeper.

Ventilation

If the air that is breathed in too many bedrooms at night could be made visible with all its impurities, the mother would resolve, with a shudder, that her child at least should never inhale such a polluted medium.

Foul air is injurious to grown persons, but it is absolutely poisonous to the sensitive organization of a child. Air that has once been breathed is unfit to be taken into the lungs again. It is laden with waste matter and has lost its oxygen, the life-giving principle. If the outside air does not enter in a steady stream, the pure air shut up in the room is exhausted in a very short time, and then nothing remains but the vitiated air to be rebreather. Lighted lamps and gas burners consume a large amount of oxygen.

Everyone acknowledges this, yet not one in twenty provides for the regular admission of pure air into the room where the baby lies asleep.

We cannot say "open the window" and dispose of the problem in this easy fashion. It must be admitted at the outset that it is difficult one, but mother love can solve it, as it does so many others.

The point is, how to keep the room filled with pure air without chilling the atmosphere and making a draught. In warm summer weather the windows can be thrown wide open and no one suffers. Even then a light screen should surround the baby's crib, and an extra covering be at hand to draw over him in the early morning.

The temperature should not be allowed to fall below 60°F, and during the greater part of the year this means that some artificial heat must be maintained to counteract the coolness of the fresh air.

When the house is heated by a furnace this is easily managed; in other circumstances, a fire in the stove, or oil stove, must not be grudged. Gas stoves are very objectionable in bedrooms, as they consume a great quantity of oxygen and give off deleterious fumes.

Having arranged to warm the fresh air, it must be admitted through a guarded window, not to create a draught. The simplest way is to lower the window from the top, or, if that sass does not let down, to open at the bottom for about four inches and take a strip of flannel over the opening. A light wooden frame, covered with flannel, may be made to fit the opening and it is easily put in and taken out. A stream of fresh air rushes in where the upper and under sashes are separated, and if the opening is at the top warm, impure air finds its way out there.

When a room smells close to anyone entering it from the outside air, it is not properly ventilated. Many persons have a horror of night air, but no one has a private receptacle which it can fill with fresh dry air to last until the sun rises again. As the children, in common with everyone else, have to breathe night air at night, let it at least be pure.

NECESSITY OF SLEEP

There is no one thing that is more conducive to a child's well-being than plenty of sleep. The warmth of it disturbs the delicate nervous system, upsets the digestion and prevents proper physical development.

It is cruel to waken a baby except for nourishment, and if it is sleeping very soundly it is better to wait for an hour beyond the appointed time, hoping that the waking will occur naturally. To take up a baby to exhibit it is an invasion to its rights that should not be tolerated for a moment.

When the darling has ceased to be a novelty, and it is earnestly desired that it may sleep while the mother is busy, it will have lost the good habits it tried to practice until it was rudely disturbed and will not be anxious to find them again.

Sleep is a positive necessity to the growing boy and girl, and yet how hard it is to send them to bed. They need ten hours, from 9:00 PM to 7:00 AM, until they are well grown sixteen or seventeen, at least.

Many girls are said to break down from over-study who could have graduated without difficulty if they had proper food and a sufficient amount of sleep.

Children should not be wakened in the morning. If they are in bed in time to obtain the measure of sleep that nature requires it will not be necessary. They should be ready to spring up fresh and vigorous, rested from the fatigue of yesterday, ready for whatever today may bring.

It has often been remarked that little children are always ready to get up in the morning, while older ones are usually reluctant to do so. If the seniors had spent an equal number of hours in bed, or at least a sufficiently long time to become thoroughly rested, they too would be satisfied and not feel the need of more sleep, which makes them so unwilling to be disturbed.

A child from one to three years old should have a nap in the morning and afternoon. These should be continued as long as the child can be persuaded to sleep in the day. The afternoon nap is especially important; the child gets tired and cross towards evening if it is missed.

IIMPORTANCE OF SEPARATE BEDS

Two children should not be allowed to sleep in the same bed; one or other will suffer from the contact. It is a serious error to permit a child to sleep with an adult, particularly an elderly person. It is not fully understood why the association should be injurious, but it does affect the vitality of the child.

THE BABY'S TOILET
CHAPTER XI

THE BABY'S BASKET

Low Baskets

A pretty basket to hold the requisites for the baby's toilet is indispensable and usually no little thought and care is expanded upon it. A flat wicker one is used for the purpose, either round, square or oval in shape, about twenty-two inches long and with the sides three to four inches high.

This can be covered with glazed cambric of any color preferred. It is a French fancy to have blue for a boy and pink for a girl, but pale primrose yellow, delicate green, or crimson in winter, look equally well. Plain, figured, or dotted muslin is fulled over the cambric, with a deep ruffle of the same around the edge trimmed with narrow lace. A piece of cardboard is cut to fit the bottom of the basket and covered with cambric and muslin. Two small pin cushions and two little bags of the same materials are fastened to the sides, ornamented with tiny bows of ribbon.

Muslin decorations always grow limp in a short time and it is more sensible to choose a wicker basket with an open edge through which ribbon of the proper width can be woven and ornamented here and there with bows. The bottom may be fitted with a sheet of cardboard covered with a thin layer of wadding sprinkled with sachet powder and over that India or China silk, either fulled a little and caught through the cardboard or put on plain. The pin cushions and bags may be of the same material, fastened to the sides of the basket with ribbon drawn through and tied on the outside. Chintz can be used instead of silk.

Standard Baskets

High baskets standing on a tripod are pretty. They can be treated with the same way and have a broad ribbon tied where the legs cross.

Hampers

A wicker hamper will hold much more than the ordinary basket. One costs about five dollars and a half untrimmed. It has a tray to hold the articles required for the toilet; pockets and pin cushions may be fastened to it. It may be lined or not as preferred and covered with muslin or silk. It looks very

Elizabeth Robinson Scovil *The Care of Children*

well with the broad ribbon crossing the cover diagonally, with a bow at each end, or arranged in two triangles crossing one another, with bows where they intersect.

When the wicker basket is not trimmed it is sometimes gilded and painted white, or red, with touches of gold, and varnished. This is a good device when the basket has done duty before and grown a little shabby in the service.

If there is no cover it is well to make one of any pretty material that can be washed, to throw over it when not in use.

THE CONTENTS

The basket must contain a powder box and puff. The former may be silver or any one of the pretty decorated ones that are perhaps even more suitable. The box is not nearly as important as the powder, which must be fine and soft. Any good toilet powder will answer; the cheaper ones sold under that name are to be suspected. Fine French chalk scented with a little powdered orris root is inexpensive and perfectly safe.

It is well to have a little china, glass or porcelain box of Vaseline.

There must be a cake of ivory soap in a celluloid or silver soap box. It is very important not to use a cheap scented soap for the delicate skin of a baby. There is no particular virtue in Castile soap, which has long been consecrated to this purpose.

A little brush and tiny comb make a pretty gift for a baby, but only the brush is needed at first. It must be a very soft as the little head does not well bear being irritated with stiff brushes bristles.

A wide-mouthed bottle of powdered borax and one of precipitated fuller's earth should be in readiness but need not be in the basket.

There should be a bunch of absorbent cotton in one pocket and an old pocket handkerchief in the other. A pair of blunt scissors, and two or three yards of soft twine may be laid in the basket when it is used for the first time. One cushion must be filled with large, and the other with small safety pins, as a common pin should never be put into a baby's clothes.

The garments that will be required for the first dressing may be laid in readiness in the basket. A band, a shirt, a flannel slip, one of the plain night slips, a napkin, a pair of socks, and a Germantown wool blanket.

Receptacles for Clothings

A chiffonier, or modern high bureau, with many shallow drawers, is a very convenient receptacle for the baby's wardrobe. A delicate fragrance ought to linger about the dainty clothing; and violet always seems to be the most appropriate odor. Sachets can be laid amongst the little garments, or a stiff piece of paper, or thin cardboard, cut to fit exactly the bottom of the drawer, a split sheet of wadding tacked on it, thickly sprinkled with violet powder covered with the other half of the sheet, and then with silk, or any material desired. The contents of the drawer will always be fragrant and not overpoweringly so.

A trunk, a large wooden box, treated in the same way, neatly lined, the top being stuffed, and the whole covered with chintz like and ottoman, is a substitute not to be despised, and makes it convenient receptacle for the napkins which often overflow a shallow drawer.

The Carriage

A young baby does not require a carriage, as it should be carried in the arms until at least two months old. The warmth and gentle motion, free from jolts and jars, are better for it than the uncertainties of a carriage, unless it is under experienced guidance.

In purchasing a carriage the money should be expended for good workmanship, smooth-running gear and stability of frame, rather than for a fine parasol, or handsome upholstering.

The wicker ones are, on the whole, the most satisfactory, and those with a hood of the same material look well longer than those with shades of less durable material.

When a parasol becomes shabby it can be recovered at a moderate expense. Lace covers can be bought which conceal the ravages of time and, as they can be washed, are easily made fresh when soiled.

A nurse maid never seems to remember that the parasol is adjustable, and is intended to shield the baby from the wind and protect the eyes from the sun. A touch will bring it into a position where it will be useful, but often during the whole time the baby is out it remains unchanged, sun and wind having it all their own way with the baby's face.

A carriage should be rolled smoothly and carefully lifted over curb stones. If mothers fully realized the risk of entrusting a baby in a carriage to an inexperienced, and sometimes untrustworthy nurse girl, they surely would hesitate to do it.

A baby's bones are not easily broken but, being much softer than an adult's, they are easily bent. A bounce, hard jolt, may do irretrievable mischief to the tender spine; a fall may render life a burden in all the years to come.

While the baby is young, it must lie flat in the carriage with a pillow as a bed. When old enough to sit up it should be carefully fastened in with one of the patent straps that render falling out almost impossible, unless the carriage is overturned. In this case the back must be comfortably supported with pillows.

A carriage blanket may be crocheted, or knitted in one color. An eiderdown or Jersey flannel blanket looks well in cool weather, or one of the pretty silk striped rugs that can be bought for the purpose.

In summer, pongee silk makes a serviceable covering. Any pretty silk may be used with a cambric lining. Fine flannel with a spray embroidered on it looks well, but soils easily. Some of the stouter linen materials, bound with braid and with the monogram worked in the center, are useful, as they can be washed. A blanket should be large enough to be well tucked in at foot and sides.

BATHS
CHAPTER XII

THE BATH TUB

A basin holds sufficient water for the baby's bath during the first few weeks. After that, an oval tin tub makes a good bathtub. When water is precious or has to be carried a long distance, a tin hat bath is the most economical. It is shaped like a large round hat, the crown containing the water. When there is a bathroom, the baby enjoys the large tub as soon as she is old enough to appreciate it.

A folding bathtub, made of heavy, flexible rubber cloth fastened to a frame, can be purchased for about five dollars. It is convenient where economy is space is an object, as it can be folded up when not in use.

China basins can be purchased with a division in the middle, one side for warm and the other for cooler water, or one for plain and the other for a scented water to finish the bath, but they are not of much practical use. They also come with wooden stands that hold the pitcher, soap dish, etc., as well.

WASH CLOTHS

These are much more satisfactory than sponges, and should be made of soft linen; part of an old napkin answers very well. It is better to ravel the edges with the fringe and overcast them than to hem them.

For older children they may be knitted of white knitting cotton or large needles to make them loose and soft, or made of a square of Turkish toweling.

CARE OF THE SPONGES

It spoils the sponge to put soap on it. It should be rinsed and clear water, squeezed dry it after using, and hung in the sun when it is convenient, or where it will dry rapidly. It is said that when a sponge becomes slimy from long use, it may be restored by boiling it in water containing a few drops of ammonia, or a little washing soda. A sponge is a source of danger unless it is kept perfectly clean. It affords a good hiding-place for poisonous germs, and it is much safer to use a washcloth.

Elizabeth Robinson Scovil *The Care of Children*

TOWELS

It is difficult to get new towels that are soft enough for the baby's first bath. They are best made of the unworn parts of an old tablecloth. If they cannot be obtained, cotton or linen diaper washed several times until the stiffness is entirely gone, makes a tolerable substitute.

Toweling can be purchased by the yard and hemmed at a cheaper rate than the finished towel can be bought. In purchasing these, it is better to avoid the fringed ones as the fringe is apt to wear off. They can be had either hemstitched or finished to imitate a hem with bands of color above it and these are very durable.

Turkish towels make the best bath towels for older children and can be had in various degrees of roughness, either fringed, or by the yard.

A separate towel should be kept for the face and hands. Towels should be changed frequently. It is not well for the children's sake to allow them to become too soiled. Each child should have his own towel.

LAP PADS

It is convenient to have a lap pad to hold the baby on when it is lifted from the tub. It should be about three-quarters of a yard long by half a yard wide. A bag is made of gray, or any pretty striped flannel, trimmed with a ruffle, if desired, and to which the pad is slipped. This is merely a piece of rubber cloth, cut to fit the bag and can be easily taken out to be dried and disinfected.

The pad is also useful to put under the baby when it is laid on the bed for a few minutes, or to place on a visitor's lap for fear of accidents. It can have strings on one side to tie around the mother's waist to prevent it from slipping when in use.

THE FIRST BATH

A baby ought not to be plunged in the water until it is at least a month old. It has been accustomed to a temperature about 99°F. We consider 80°F hot for a room, nearly twenty degrees colder. No doubt, the exposure of washing is responsible for many of the bronchial affections, colds in the head, etc., that affect and sometimes prove fatal to little babies.

The first bath should be given on the mother's lap, the baby lying between the folds of a blanket. A small, soft, old one is the best for this purpose; if one is not to be had, a new crib blanket should be provided or two yards of eiderdown flannel.

If there is much sebaceous or cheese-like matter adhering to the skin, as there is apt to be in some parts, it should be rubbed with Vaseline or a little olive oil. The water should be comfortably warm, the cloth squeezed out of it and the little white soap rubbed on it. The nurse's hand holding the cloth should be passed under the blanket and a part of the surface of the body washed and dried with pats of a soft towel before proceeding to the next portion. A baby's skin is so delicate it should never be rubbed except on the gentlest manner. It is not absolutely essential that every particle of the sebaceous matter should be removed at the first bath.

After being dried, the baby should be lightly powdered from head to foot, particularly under the arms and wherever folds of skin come together, as in the thighs.

Every time a napkin is removed the parts should be wiped with a moist, warm cloth, dried and powdered. Attention to the simple precaution will prevent chafing.

SPONGE BATHS

It takes only a very few moments to give a child a sponge bath, either in the morning or evening, and it should be done not less frequently than every other day, if it is impossible to give it oftener.

A bathtub is not necessary. The water should be cool but not icy cold. The face and neck should be washed first, then the arms, next the body and last the legs and feet. The sponging should be quickly and lightly done with the cloth comfortably moist but not dripping, each part being dried before the next is wetted. It should be followed by quick rubbing of the whole body to stimulate the circulation. A delicate child can stand with the feet in warm water while the bath is being given.

The whole body should not be exposed at once, one-half being covered while the other is done. The room should be comfortably warm and draughts guarded against.

As soon as children are old enough, they should be taught to give themselves a sponge bath every morning. It removes the impurities cast out with the perspiration by the million pores of the skin, and, by invigorating the body, renders the surface less susceptible to cold. A hardy child does not take cold easily.

COLD BATHS

Little children should not be plunged into cold water. After two years of age, a cold bath of a temperature not below 60°F once or twice a week will do no harm to a vigorous child. It should never be taken immediately after eating. It is better for two hours to intervene between meal and the bath.

The test of its agreeing with the child is the reaction which follows it. If the blood is brought to the surface, the skin glows and there is a delightful sensation of tingling warmth, it has done good. When the bather looks blue and feels chilly, its you should be discontinued.

Warm Baths

Hot baths of temperature of 100°F, or above it, should not be given to children without medical advice. They are too enervating to be indulged in with impunity. The ordinary warm plunge bath should not be hotter than 95°F. When one is taken the sponge bath should, of course, be omitted for that day.

In putting a sick child who is afraid of water into a warm bath, the tub can be covered with the small, thin blanket or square of flannel, the child laid on this and gently lowered into the water.

When a child is ailing, feverish and fretful, a warm bath often gives relief. If it is the beginning of an eruptive disease, the warmth and moisture help to bring out the rash. It is always soothing and tends to induce sleep. The drying must be done under a blanket.

Saltwater Baths

Saltwater baths are especially invigorating to delicate children; they often derive more benefit from them than from sea bathing, which may be too great a shock, if the child is nervous or afraid of the water.

Dissolve a quarter of a pound of rock salt in one gallon of water for a sponge bath, using the same proportion for the greater quantity required for a plunge bath. Sea water may be used when it can be procured, or sea salt, which can be purchased in boxes. The bath should always be followed by brisk rubbing.

Foot Baths

These are useful when a child has a bad cold in the head, or on the chest, or the head is hot. Place the invalid in a low chair with the feet in a tub or pail of water as hot as can be comfortably borne, enveloping pail and knees in a blanket wrapped around them. Keep up the temperature by pouring in a little hot water at the side from time to time. Mustard, about two teaspoonfuls to the gallon, can be added if more stimulation is desired.

The bath should last about ten minutes, the feet being carefully dried after it and the child put to bed. Warmer stockings than usual should be worn next day.

To give a foot bath and badly a square of rubber cloth under the sheet, put the basin on this, let the child lie on his back and drawing up the knees place the feet in the water. A blanket protects from exposure.

The Sponge Bath in Bed

Lay a folded blanket on one side of the bed and lift the child on it. Place another blanket over him and under cover of it remove the night dress. With the soft cloth wash the face and neck and dry them with a warm towel, next do the arms, then the chest. Turning the child on the side, wash the back and thighs; laying him again on the back do the legs and feet. All must be done under the blanket without exposure and each part dried before the next is wetted.

When a child is restless and feverish this will often induce sleep and reduce the temperature. The water should be cool, about 75°F, and no soap need be used.

The night dress should be warmed before it is replaced.

The Cold Pack

This is sometimes ordered by the physician when there is much fever. The bed is covered with two or three blankets, folded double, on these is laid a folded sheet wrung out of cold water; the child is placed on this and the sheets and blankets folded over him. The feet are left uncovered and the hot water bag applied to them if they grow cold. Plenty of water is given to drink. The treatment may be continued for two or three hours and is usually very comfortable, causing sleep and relieving the fever and restlessness.

In exceedingly hot weather babies who suffer much from the heat are sometimes wrapped in a wet sheet, which is kept wet for half an hour at a time. The clothing is of course removed.

The Bran Bath

In diseases of the skin rainwater should be used for bathing in the surface. If this cannot be obtained brand or starch should be used. The former is a pleasant addition to the bathwater even when its use is not absolutely necessary. It softens and is said to whiten the skin. Put a pound of brand in a bag and boil it in eight quarts of water, using the water for the bath and diluting it if necessary.

Starch Bath

Take two tablespoonfuls of starch, rub it smooth the little cold water, and add it to about two quarts of water. In diseases of the skin the drying should be accomplished by padding with a soft towel, no friction being permitted.

Elizabeth Robinson Scovil *The Care of Children*

Open Air Bathing

Sea bathing is invigorating to children if they are in a condition to bear it. There are some precautions which should be taken. An hour and a half or two hours must relapse between a meal and the bath. The child should not be permitted to stay in the water more than fifteen minutes, and often a shorter time is all that is permissible. The child should never be forced to go in when he is afraid, from a mistaken idea of making him hardy. Usually, he can be encouraged and persuaded to make the attempt and ends up liking the fun. If it is impossible to reassure him, the bath should be abandoned until he gains more confidence.

Bathing in fresh water is more apt to be injurious than in salt water, and should never be prolonged.

Not more than one bath a day should be permitted. Children who live near a lake, or other body of fresh water, like to bathe several times a day in warm weather, but dangerous results are apt to follow.

Waiting when the sun is hot is not a safe amusement. The feet are immersed in cold water, and the head, exposed to the sun's rays, is overheated, not a desirable combination of circumstances.

Necessity for Care in Bathing

Delicate children should not be washed too often. It exhausts their vitality, and is too great a drain on their recuperative powers.

A puny baby is sometimes not washed for several days after its birth, warm oil being used to rub it instead of giving it a bath. The parts particularly requiring it are cleaned from time to time with a moist cloth.

When a child cannot have a full bath, very often the body can be bathed with impunity by doing a small part each day until the whole is gone over, keeping this up systematically.

Such children should be rubbed from head to foot with a square of Turkish toweling once a day. This cleanses the skin to a certain extent, and the friction stimulates the circulation.

A girl never should be permitted to take a plunge in a bath near the menstrual period, and even cold sponge baths should be prohibited while it lasts. Careful washing with warm water is all that must be allowed.

CARE OF THE TEETH
CHAPTER XIII

TEETHING

The period of teething is always one of more or less anxiety to the mother. Even in a perfectly healthy child there is usually some disturbance of the system, although this may be very slight and never amount to actual illness.

WHEN TEETH MAY BE EXPECTED

It is difficult to say positively at what time the first teeth may be expected to appear. They may arrive as early as the fourth month, but do not usually come until the sixth or seventh and sometimes are delayed much later.

If none have come through the gums by the time the child is a year old, a physician should be consulted, as the nutrition may be faulty, or some constitutional treatment be required.

THE EARLIEST SIGNS

The gums, which have been smooth and soft though firm, begin to be a little swelled in front and the secretion of saliva increases, causing the baby to drool. This may continue for a month or two, before the teeth can be felt projecting under the edge of the gum. The child seems to find relief in biting any hard substance, although one would think the pressure on the gum would be painful.

When this stage is prolonged, the gums sometimes become very much swollen, are hot to the touch and the condition is one of so much irritation that the doctor lances them, setting the tooth free. This sometimes saves much unnecessary suffering.

ORDER OF APPEARANCE

One of the two lower middle teeth is usually the first to emerge, as the piercing of the gum by the teeth is technically called. These are followed by two corresponding upper ones, the four being known as the central incisors.

There should be a rest of about two months before the next four in each side of them appear. These are called the lateral or side incisors and the lower ones may be expected first.

When the child is about a year old, the first double teeth or interior molars should come through. These are not next the lateral incisors, but one space beyond them, room being left for the cuspid teeth, or eye or stomach teeth, as they are properly called, which do not come before the seventeenth to the twentieth month. When the child is about two years old, the posterior molars make their appearance at the back of the mouth, completing the set of first or milk teeth, twenty in number. The molars are broad on the top with a depression in the middle. The edges of the ridges come through first, occasionally creating the impression that two teeth are on the way.

The lower molars have two roots, the upper molars three and the other teeth one each.

Duration of Teething

The cutting of the first teeth is often not finished before the end of the second year, so that it lasts about eighteen months.

It is a matter of congratulation when there is a pause between the emerging of the different groups of teeth, as it gives the child time to recuperate.

The teeth are partly formed in the jaw at the time of birth and instances have been known where babies were born with them more or less developed.

Allaying the Discomfort

Water should be given freely during teething. When the gums are much inflamed, small lumps of ice may be wrapped in a piece of gauze or thin muslin and given to the child to suck. Rubbing and gums with lemon juice sometimes helps relieve the irritation.

When little ulcerated spots appear, a pinch of powdered Borax may be stirred into a small quantity of glycerin and the ulcers touched with it three or four times a day.

When the head is hot, it can be bathed in cool water.

Teething Rings

Something hard to bite upon is a necessity to the teething baby. A rubber ring is the most satisfactory, as the surface yields a little and yet is not too soft to offer the necessary resistance. Anything that the baby can lay hands on upon is carried to the mouth, and the surface that is not smooth, as well as hard, always provokes a cry of pain.

Disorders Incident to Teething—Diarrhea

The mother must be on her guard against imagining that diarrhea is always a necessary accompaniment of teething and so neglecting it.

It is a symptom of some disturbance of the digestive tract and should not be allowed to go on unchecked. While this is true, the bowels will probably be rather more relaxed than usual, but this need not cause alarm, if the character of the motions is good.

Paralysis of the legs or arms, or one of each, sometimes follows the emerging of the molar teeth. It is said to be generally temporary, lasting a few weeks only.

Convulsions are always an alarming symptom to the mother. If the gums are very hot and swollen, they should be lanced. The child should have a warm bath, as directed elsewhere, and the physician be sent for.

Rashes

These frequently appear from the irritation of the system. If there is constipation, a gentle laxative, as spice syrup or rhubarb, may be given. The eruption can be bathed in a little decarbonate of soda, baking soda, dissolved in water. This will help to relieve the itching, if this symptom is present.

The rash is usually of little importance, does not require treatment, and disappears after a time.

In warm weather, the child should spend much time in the open air and in a shady place, not be overburdened with clothes, and kept as cool as possible.

Sunshine and fresh air are especially needed when this trying period comes in winter. The nursery must be kept well-ventilated and the sunlight freely admitted.

The Second Teeth

It seems strange that the first teeth, acquired with so much difficulty, should last only a few years and then have to be replaced by a second set.

The first of the permanent teeth to appear are the four molars beyond the last molars of the temporary set. These may be looked for when the child is from five and a half to seven years old. They are often mistaken for first teeth and so do not receive the attention they require. The child should be taken to a dentist that he may be sure there is no irregularity in their position and that all is right.

Very often the advent of the second teeth is accompanied by disturbance of the digestion and general health, which is not always traced to its true cause.

In a few months the new middle incisors, or cutting teeth, push the old ones out and occupy their places. The new tooth absorbs the root of the old so that the latter are very loosely attached to the gum and often can be dislodged with the fingers alone. The upper incisors should pierce the gum outside the old ones, the lower come inside their predecessors. Sometimes a year passes before the lateral, or side incisors, follow the middle ones.

When the child is about ten the eight bicuspids, or two pointed teeth, next to the cuspid, come into view.

About two years later the two lower cuspids make their appearance, followed in from one to three years by the two upper ones.

The second molars appear from the twelfth to the fourteenth year, the third molars, or wisdom teeth, at any time after the seventeenth year, making in all thirty-two, sixteen in each jaw.

The Care of the Teeth

Teeth are so important to the comfort and health that no care and pains that can be expended upon them is too great. Frequent cleansing and particularly passing a fine thread between those sufficiently separated to permit its passage to dislodge any mischief making atom that may have found a place there, is the best preservative measure.

Rinsing the mouth with a little lime water at night removes the traces of any acid that may have been there during the day.

It is a mistaken idea that the first teeth need little or no attention. Until the child is old enough to attend to it himself, the mother should use the soft brush, at least twice a day, cleansing the teeth thoroughly.

The child should be taught to use the brush after each meal and to pass a fine thread of silk between the teeth at the same time to dislodge any particle of food or foreign matter that may be there.

This is of the greatest importance, as the comparatively trifling obstruction, if left undisturbed may cause the serious cavity.

If the teeth are properly cleansed after eating, nothing that is taken into the mouth can injure them, because it is not allowed to remain in contact with them enough to do harm.

When medicine is given, iron and acid should be taken through a glass tube.

Tooth powders are not necessary to keep the teeth in good order. Pure soft water and a brush are all sufficient if they are used with the necessary frequency. Many dentifrices do more harm than good.

A dentist should be consulted before even the first tooth is removed. If taken out too soon the jaw is permitted to contract and the tooth which comes to occupy the place is unduly crowded.

If the teeth are not perfectly even and regular the child ought to be taken to a dentist. Defects can often be remedied if attended to in time which it is impossible to rectify after years of neglect.

It is comparatively easy to straighten teeth and put them in their proper relative position while the child is young and it is wrong to permit a deformity to exist which might have been prevented if proper means had been used.

Grinding the Teeth

This is a popularly supposed to be an unfailing symptom of the pressure of worms in the intestines. It is usually noticed in sleep, and is sometimes an indication of disease of the brain. Usually, however, it proceeds from that fruitful source of the ills of childhood, a disordered digestion. It frequently occurs when there is diarrhea and is generally only temporary, disappearing when the cause is removed. If it persists the doctor should be consulted.

Toothache

This is a common affliction when the teeth decay. If there is a cavity, a drop of carbolic acid, creosote, or oil of cloves, put on a cottonwool and pressed into the into the hole, often gives ease.

When no opening can be detected dissolve a teaspoonful of powdered alum in sweet spirits of niter and bathe the gum on each side of the tooth with the mixture.

If there are shooting pains that cannot be traced to any one tooth, neuralgia may be at the bottom of the mischief, and quinine, or some other tonic, be needed, with more stimulating and nutritious food.

Very often extraction, or at least treatment by the dentist, is the only thing that will bring permanent relief.

CARE OF THE EYES
CHAPTER XIV

THE EYES

A defect in sight is such a grievous affliction in later life to a person burdened with it that the care of the eyes in children becomes a matter of the first importance.

It is interesting to the mother to know that the color of a baby's eyes is not fixed until after it is six weeks or two months old. They may change to a lighter or a darker shade.

Ophthalmia of the New Born

The slightest redness, or swelling, about the eyes of a young infant should receive immediate attention. It is accompanied by a slight discharge which, if neglected, may cause loss of sight.

This is so important that in France a nurse is obliged by law to report to a competent medical authority any affection of the eyes of a newborn child.

The first symptoms may appear when the baby is two to three days old.

Perfect cleanliness is the remedy, not allowing the discharge to accumulate on the cornea, or transparent covering of the eye. If this is permitted, an ulcer may form, penetrate the cornea, and produce blindness.

The lower lid must be gently drawn down at the outer corner, and tepid water put in with a dropper, or small syringe, thoroughly washing the whole surface. The doctor will probably order a slightly astringent wash. If the discharge adheres to the eyelids, they can be touched with Vaseline, or a drop or two of pure oil.

The eyes sometimes require washing as often as once in fifteen minutes, the frequency depending on the amount of the secretion. The nurse is responsible for the child's sight, and this thought should make her faithful to her duty.

The disease is very infectious. The nurse must carefully guard her own eyes and those of the mother. Pieces of soft cotton should be used to cleanse and wipe the eyes, and immediately burned. The nurse must disinfect her hands after touching the eyes or she may convey the infection by means of her fingertips.

SHADING THE EYES

A young baby's eyes should not be exposed to strong light. This does not mean that the sunlight must be kept out of the room, but that the baby's eyes must be shaded from its direct rays. The canopy of the crib, or a screen, should protect them. It is equally injurious to let the gas, or any artificial light, shine directly on them.

Older children should be taught to guard the eyes carefully, particularly when studying at night.

A paper shade over the eyes is often a great relief.

In climates where there is much snow, the sun shining on the dazzling white surface is very trying. Smoked or colored glasses should be worn if this strain causes stinging, or inflammation of the eyes.

Wind is very injurious to weak eyes, and they should be protected from it by glasses.

TESTING THE EYES

Many persons never discover that their vision is not normal until some accidental occurrence reveals to them the fact that they do not see as well as their fellow beings.

Having always been accustomed to a limited range of sight, they do not realize that others have a wider field. Their own defect of vision, whatever it may be, is a part of their daily experience, and unless the difference between themselves and their more gifted companions is forced upon them, they do not recognize it.

Children are often unjustly blamed for being stupid, or inattentive, when the truth is they cannot see clearly what they are required to understand.

The mother should try to ascertain the amount of vision possessed by her child. She can find which details of a picture he can see at various distances; whether he can distinguish the faces of passersby on the opposite side of the street, and before he goes to school what ability he has to read words and figures removed from him, as on a blackboard.

The eyes should be tested separately by covering first one and then the other. If there is any doubt as to the site being perfectly normal they should be examined by a specialist.

DEFECTS OF VISION

The most common defects in vision are short sight, long sight, and astigmatism.

Elizabeth Robinson Scovil *The Care of Children*

Short Sight

When the child seems to have difficulty in distinguishing objects at a distance, short sight should be suspected, and the eyes examined by an oculist. A child between eight and twelve years old should be able to read ordinary print with the book held at a distance of thirteen inches from the eye.

Short sight can be corrected by proper glasses, and even very little children can wear them.

Short sight may be produced where it does not exist naturally by overstraining the eyes, as in reading by a bad light.

Long Sight

The child is unable to use his eyes to see objects at a short distance without straining them he cannot accommodate the sight easily to a short range and the effort to do so often causes headache. The eyes feel strained, and the letters look blurred. Pressure is sometimes made with the hand, as it feels as it gives the feeling of relief, or the eyes are often closed to rest them.

If the defect is not remedied by proper glasses, it may produce a permanent squint.

Astigmatism is caused by a defect in the curve of the cornea or front of the eyeball. While objects can be seen, their outline is blurred and there is a certain indistinctness about everything. It can be entirely corrected by glasses, when it is the only defect in the eye, and usually materially helped by them in any case.

The eyes can be tested only by an oculus, as he has the proper apparatus for doing so. When any defect is known or suspected, the child should at once have the best advice obtainable.

Squinting

When the squint is first observed, the well eye should be covered for a short interval several times a day to oblige the other one to do its duty properly. Much may be done by proper treatment under the direction of a competent oculus. If the squint is for is of long standing, an operation will probably be necessary.

The Consequences of Eye Strain

An undue strain upon the eyes is the cause of many ailments and diseases that apparently have little or no connection with them.

Headache is one of the most common and obvious. Many nervous affections, as chorea or Saint Vitus' dance, are caused or aggravated by disease of the eyes.

Indigestion, want of appetite and the general malaise which we sometimes term being out of sorts, occasionally have the same origin.

Often proper glasses will cure when drugs and dieting have been tried in vain. This should be borne in mind when seeking for the cause of a child's indisposition.

Conjunctivitis

This is an inflammation of the delicate membrane covering the white of the eye, or the conjunctiva. One form is known as "pink eye". The eye is so delicate that a physician should always be consulted when it is affected, as it is not safe to treat it with home remedies. The utmost that should be ventured on is to wash it frequently with boiled water which has stood until it is tepid; or, a solution of boracic acid of fifteen grains to the ounce. When the eye is intolerant of light, dark glasses should be worn until advice can be obtained.

Poultices should never be applied to the eyes, nor any soft, moist application that will act in the same manner.

When cold is ordered, it is best to have several small squares of linen laid on a lump of ice, putting one on the eye at a time and changing it as soon as it begins to dry. If it is simply to subdue inflammation, the pieces may be used again. When there is a discharge from the eye, each piece should be burned after it is removed.

Nourishing food, fresh air, and a tonic, as iron or quinine, are necessary to effect a cure, if the child is in a reduced condition.

Studying at Night

When eyes and brain are tired, it is cruel to urge them to further exertion. The study of books, especially with younger children, should not be required except during school hours.

If it cannot be avoided in the case of older ones, it should not be begun immediately after tea, and two periods of half an hour each should be insisted upon, instead of a whole hour being given to it at once. Studies that require more than an hour of labor in the evening should be discontinued. There ought to be an interval of half an hour between putting away the books and bedtime.

Artificial Light

If work must be done at night, it is very important that a proper light should be provided to do it by.

A flickering, unsteady flame ruins the eyes.

Elizabeth Robinson Scovil *The Care of Children*

A good lamp, of the kind known as "student lamp", is, perhaps, the best. At least, the lamp should have a shade — green lined with white is the most restful to the eyes — to throw the light downward on the book.

It should be placed at a slightly higher level than the head of the student, but not far enough away to diminish the brilliancy of the light.

The heat from the lamp brought close to the eyes is very injurious to them, and particularly when it stands directly in front of the face and only a few inches above it.

In working by daylight, the child should, if possible, sit with the left side towards the light; he never should face a window.

The most eminent authorities on the eye consider that bad light is one of the most common causes of near sight, as the eye is under a perpetual strain.

Styes

These are little tumors which appear on the edge of the eyelid and are often troublesome and painful. When they first appear their progress may be stopped by touching them with collodion, which can be obtained in bottles from the apothecary.

Bathing them with a warm saturated solution of boracic acid often gives relief when they are further advanced. If there is much inflammation, pieces of cotton rung out of hot water may be held over them for a few minutes at a time.

They are sometimes caused by constipation, and if there is a succession of them a tonic and attention to the diet are needed.

Foreign Bodies in the Eye

When a foreign substance gets in the eye the child should if possible be prevented from rubbing the lid, as that only presses it further into the eyeball. The first thing to do is to part the lids with a thumb and finger as widely as possible; often the sudden gush of tears will bring away the offending particle. Sometimes rubbing the other eye will stimulate the secretion.

Blowing the nose may carry it into the tear duct, which opens into the nose from the inner corner of the eye.

If these methods fail, the lower lid should be drawn down and carefully examined for the cause of the trouble. If not there, a slate pencil can be pressed against the upper lid and the edge rolled up over it by holding the eyelashes. Often the spec will be found under it and can be gently wiped out with the handkerchief.

The eye may be syringed with warm water, using a small glass syringe, or a medicine dropper.

If none of these means are effectual, the physician must be applied to.

When the eye is burnt with the strong acid it must be bathed with the weak solution of baking soda in water.

If an alkali, as lime, is the agent, very weak vinegar and water, or sugar and water can be used.

In either case it is a great relief to apply Vaseline or castor oil liberally to both lids, so that it will spread over the eye and soothe the inflammation. These emollients may be used whenever the eyes are seriously inflamed. No one who has not experienced it can know the delicious sensation of velvet like softness when they are brought in contact with the painful eye.

A feeling like grains of sand in the eyes indicates inflammation.

Color Blindness

Some persons do not possess the power of distinguishing certain colors apart. They are most apt to confuse green and red, although these seem so different to the normal eye.

A book with a bright red cover was pointed out to a person with this defect; very little difference could be detected between it and one of a dark green hue that lay beside it. A sofa covering of stripes of crimson and olive green presented an almost uniform gray tint, there being a slight difference in intensity of color, or depth of shade, between the two.

It is by this difference in the shade that children, who have this defect, must be taught to distinguish colors. The mother may do much by careful training. Teaching them to select and sort strands of different colored wools is one of the methods. Counters of various hues may be used for the same purpose. Scraps of silk, worsted or cotton materials may be utilized, provided exactly the same fabric can be found in the requisite colors.

It must be by the variation in intensity of tone and not by any accidental difference of shape, size or texture that the child recognizes the object, if the process of sorting it is to educate the eye.

Color blindness is a disadvantage in many trades and professions, and every effort should be made to atone for the deficiency as far as possible.

CARE OF THE EARS
CHAPTER XV

THE CONSTRUCTION OF THE EAR

The ear is a complicated piece of mechanism, as wonderful in construction as the eye. It consists of three divisions, or chambers. The inner ear is solidly lodged in one of the bones of the skull. The middle ear contains a chain of small bones by which the vibrations of the air are conveyed to the nerve of hearing, and so to the brain. It is connected with the throat, or rather with the back of the mouth, by a passage called the eustachian tube. When this tube is ulcerated, as it sometimes is in scarlet fever, the hearing is impaired. Finally, there is an outer ear with the little canal leading towards the middle ear, and closed at that end by a membrane forming one side of the "drum of the ear", as it is popularly called.

It will be seen in syringing the ear the fluid can only go as far as this membrane and cannot penetrate the middle ear.

In laying a baby down care should be taken that the ear lies flat, and is not turned under.

PROMINENT EARS

Many mothers are distressed because their children's ears stand out from the head. This physical peculiarity cannot be fully overcome, because it is due to the construction of the ear, but it may be lessened by persistent general pressure if it is begun early enough.

EAR CAPS

Caps are sold for the purpose of confining the ears close to the head. One can be made by taking a straight strip of muslin, or net, about three inches wide from the front piece, holding it over the ears and fitting to it two straps, one crossing the nape of the neck, and the other few inches higher. The extra fullness where the strip crosses the head on top is taken up and strings are added.

FLOPPY EARS

When the upper part of the ear lacks firmness and falls over, it should be bathed in salt and water twice a day, being rubbed and manipulated at the same time.

Keeping the Ears Clean

Every fold and crease of the outside ear should receive attention, but it must be done gently with warm water and a soft cloth. This is the only means needed to cleanse sufficiently the inner passage. It is an old saying that nothing smaller than the elbow should be put in the ear. This rather startling statement excludes the hairpins and other small hard instruments which are frequently used to remove wax. A hasty push might do a serious harm to the membrane, or to the delicate lining of the tube, so is best not to run the risk. A washcloth doubled and twisted to a point is all sufficient as only the opening of the canal should be cleansed.

Wax

Wax, or cerumen, as it is technically called, is a secretion prepared by nature for a special purpose. It moistens the passage, makes the lining soft and pliable, keeps particles of dust and foreign matter floating in the air from entering, and by its bitterness and oily nature prevents insects from straying into the opening. When it becomes dry it rolls into little crumbs and comes away naturally, and it is these only, lying in sight, which should be removed and washing.

Occasionally the wax forms in hard masses, interfering with the hearing. It is difficult for anyone not a surgeon to determine when this has occurred.

The ear may be gently syringed with warm water; if this does not remove it, it will have to be done with surgical instruments.

Protecting the Ears

In young children the ears should be covered in cold weather when they are out of doors. Being more sensitive than those of an adult, inflammation is more easily exited and dreaded carache set up.

Boxing the Ears

It is criminal to strike a child a blow on the ear. The air is driven with such force against the memory membrane that it may rupture. Should this occur the opening of the ears should be stopped with a plug of cotton. The injury may heal of itself if it is not meddled with. Pulling the ears may cause serious inflammation, the impulse being transmitted from the outer ear to the more sensitive parts.

Earache

Dry heat is the safest application — a hot water bag, a hop pillow, made by sowing dry hops in a bag and heating them in the oven, or a warm iron wrapped in flannel.

Elizabeth Robinson Scovil *The Care of Children*

If the nose is stopped, clearing it by means of sneezing brought about by a few grains of snuff, or pepper, will sometimes relieve the pain.

The best authorities agree that poultices, or any internal application to the ear, as hot oil, etc., may produce serious results.

Sometimes the mild mustard paste, one part mustard to six of flour, placed directly behind the ear, will give relief. It must not be left on too long for fear of blistering.

When a young baby has earache it presses the side of the head against a mother's breast, and cries incessantly until the pain is relieved.

Older babies, who cannot speak, will often hold the hand pressed against the ear, or pull at it to show it is hurting them.

Foreign Body in the Ear

The mother may remember for her comfort that the presence of a foreign body in the ear for a short time will not do any harm. It cannot penetrate to the brain because the passage is closed at the end by the membrane. There is therefore opportunity to try quietly to extract it. If it was small enough to go in, it is small enough to come out again.

If the visitor is an insect, make the child lay his head on the table with the injured ear uppermost and fill the tube with warm water or oil. The insect may float to the surface and then can be lifted out. Turn the head over and most of the oil will escape or can be absorbed by a plug of cotton wool.

Very gentle syringing will probably remove any hard substance, as a button or a bead. The head can be held with the affected ear downwards over a basin, the nozzle of the syringe being directed towards the upper part of the opening.

Moisture will make a pea or bean swell, and only increase the size, so it is best to take the child to a surgeon and not attempt to remove it by home treatment.

Holding the affected ear downwards and gently striking the opposite side of the head or shaking the head, may dislodge it, but it should not be poked at.

Syringing the Ear

This must be done in the gentlest manner not to force the stream of water too violently against the tightly structured membrane.

A glass syringe with a blunt nozzle is the best instrument to use. An ordinary bulb syringe can be made to answer the purpose if it is used with care. Select the largest nozzle; do not place it too close to the opening of the passage that there may be plenty of room for the water to escape freely. Squeeze the bulb very slowly and with only sufficient force to send the stream of water into the ear.

This treatment is often ordered by the physician when there is disease of the ear and it is well to know exactly how it should be done.

Diseases of the Ear

In all cases where there is a discharge from the ear the child should have competent medical advice. If a child is habitually inattentive when spoken to in an ordinary tone of voice the mother should suspect deafness and take pains to find out if he can hear single words spoken at a distance of three to four feet from the ear. If he cannot, or there is any evidence of impaired hearing, and aurist should be consulted if possible, or in any case the family physician.

It is said that children who breathe through the mouth are always threatened with carache and deafness. It is worth some trouble on the part of the parents to see that the habit of breathing through the nose is established. The nasal passages should be treated if any obstruction there prevents a full breath being taken through them.

Children subject to carache should not be allowed to bathe in cold water, nor to dive underwater. They should be warmly clothed and the feet protected with special care.

CARE OF THE HAIR
CHAPTER XVI

BRUSHING

Nothing improves the hair more than systematic brushing. A natural oil is secreted at the roots which, if it is not present in sufficient quantity, keeps the hair soft and glossy. Regular brushing morning and evening stimulates these glands and causes them to perform their function better. This is often the only remedy needed when the hair is harsh and dry.

COMBING

A comb is only required to part the hair, or to smooth it when it is tangled. Scraping the scalp with a fine comb should be avoided as it injures the skin and aggravates the dandruff it is used to remove.

CURLING

When a child's hair does not curl naturally, it is most sensible not to try to effect this result by artificial means.

The tight ringlets that used to be thought so beautiful, are no longer in fashion; soft, loose curls are all that is desired.

Twisting the hair into hard knobs at night breaks and injuries it, beside being very uncomfortable to the sleeper. Oily applications are not recommended for the hair. Used occasionally and for a special purpose, they may be permitted. It is said the following recipe will make the hair curl: olive oil, four ounces; oil of Origanum (wild marjoram), sixty drops; oil of rosemary, twenty drops. Shake well before using and apply frequently.

CRIMPING

If it is desired to crimp the hair, part it in the back, drawing each division well to the side, dampen it slightly and braid it loosely. By this arrangement the child is not forced to lie on the hard ridges at night.

TANGLES

When long hair has been neglected it will be very difficult to disentangle it. Time and patience are necessary, as only a portion could be done at once. The tangles can be saturated with alcohol, or, if this fails, with olive oil. Beginning at the ends work patiently until one lock is free. The ends must be held tightly near the head to prevent the painful pulling of the scalp.

CUTTING

Hair grows from the roots and dies at the ends. When they are split they must be clipped. It was an old superstition that hair always must be cut when the moon was on the increase, or it would not grow again.

When the hair is thin and scanty it often benefits it to cut it close to the head. A stimulating lotion should be applied at the same time.

When a boy has pretty, curling hair, it is always a trial to the mother to cut it off. The sacrifice should be made when he is promoted to trousers. Long curls look out of place with the boy's dress and are sure to expose the wearer to taunts from his companions that are hard to bear.

If a child who has unusually long, thick hairs suffers from headache, or complains frequently of its weight, not of the trouble of having it dressed, it should be removed.

BANGS

Bangs are not objectionable, if they are not too long. They should not be curled or crimped, particularly in girls, as it is important that the front hair should not be injured.

Keeping the hair short for any length of time does not interfere with its future growth, but rather promotes it.

In arranging the hair, it should not be tied back too tightly to bring a strain upon the scalp.

Wearing the hair over the forehead does not make it grow lower, as is sometimes imagined. There is a certain line in every individual beyond which the hair follicles or roots do not develop, and no training will make them so.

THIN HAIR

In some families the hair is naturally abundant and beautiful, in others it is thin and harsh, or scanty and very fine, without apparent cause. These idiosyncrasies must be taken into consideration.

Persistent brushing does much to stimulate the growth of the hair. If an application is desired, the following formula is a good one. It must be prepared by a druggist:

- sulphate of quinine, one drachm;
- aromatic sulphoric acid, sufficient to dissolve the quinine;
- tincture of cantharides, three drachms;

Elizabeth Robinson Scovil *The Care of Children*

- glycerin, one ounce;
- rose water, three ounces;
- distilled water, sufficient to make eight ounces.

Apply every other night for two weeks, rubbing it in thoroughly.

When the hair is very thin, it is best to keep it cut close to the head. If the hair falls out in the patches, there is probably ringworm or some disease of the scalp. Attention to the diet and perhaps a tonic is needed.

Harsh Hair

This is the result of in insufficient secretion of the natural oil, which renders the hair soft and glossy.

Frequent brushing is still the best remedy. A little pure olive oil or fresh castor oil, scented with essence of verbena, can be thoroughly rubbed into the scalp two or three times a week. The rubbing probably does as much good as the oil.

Splitting at the Ends

As has been said, hair grows from the head outward, so that splitting at the ends is not of much consequence except as showing that the hair is not as moist as it should be. The ends can be clipped and a little oil applied to the scalp, if the hair is particularly dry.

Dandruff

This affection is not the result of a want of neatness, but of a disease of the scalp which causes the skin to come off and dry scales or flakes. It requires stimulating treatment. Compound camphor liniment rubbed in each night for a week and a repeated when necessary is effectual.

The hair should be washed once a week to remove the accumulation of dried skin, but the use of a fine comb should be avoided.

Special attention should be paid to the diet of the children who have dandruff, or in whom the natural secretion of oil is deficient. They need cream, butter and any form of fat they can be induced to take.

Washing the Hair

Too frequent washing of the head is injurious to the hair and tends to make it dry and harsh. Unless there is a special reason for its not its being done more frequently, once a month is sufficient, if it has daily a thorough brushing in the interval. The parting of the hair about the temples can be washed with a soft cloth weekly as the skin there is more exposed to dust.

A pinch of borax or a few drops of ammonia can be added to the water. Care must be taken not to put in too much, as the alkali removes the oil from the hair and makes it harsh for a time.

A yoke of an egg lightly beaten and well rubbed in is an excellent application to cleanse the hair. It must be washed off with Ivory soap and water. When the hair is naturally soft and glossy the white of an egg may be used to advantage in cleaning it.

PARASITES

Children sometimes become contaminated with these troublesome pests at school. When there is a reason to fear that there has been exposure, a careful examination must be made, particularly if scratching shows that there is any irritation. They increase with great rapidity.

A thorough application of kerosene oil is the safest remedy and a most effectual one. Various parasiticides can be used, but they are all poisons, while the oil is harmless.

After saturating the hair with it, a good washing in soap and water is in order. When the hair is cleansed, soaking it in vinegar will prevent the nits or eggs from developing. A close watch should be kept that the intruders do not return.

COLOR OF THE HAIR

The hair which covers the head at birth always drops out and the new growth is of a different texture and perhaps color.

It has a tendency to grow darker with age and often after seven years there is a decided change in the color. The pretty flaxen locks disappear, when the hair is light, given place to some shade of brown. The alteration in dark hair is of course not so marked.

Any attempt to alter the color of the hair by chemical means is sure to end disastrously. Nature tones it to suit the complexion and interference with her handiwork seldom results in improvement.

Red hair, which is often a trial to its possessor, is held in high esteem by artists. It usually accompanies a beautiful complexion which, if not perfect in childhood, may become so later on.

Elizabeth Robinson Scovil *The Care of Children*

Superfluous Hair

In children in whom the growth of hair is vigorous it sometimes appears in places where it is not desired, as on the face, though this is not as common in childhood as an adult life.

This superfluous hair can be removed by the use of strong alkalis, but they cannot be applied at home with safety.

It is said that the only effectual means of preventing a recurrence of the growth is to have it exterminated by means of electrolysis. The hair follicles are transfixed with fine needles connected with a battery and a current of electricity accomplishes their destruction.

Shaving it with the razor, or plucking out each hair singly with tweezers, only makes them grow stronger and harsher.

CARE OF THE NAILS
CHAPTER XVII

THE NAILS

Well-kept nails are an ornament to the hand. If children are early trained to bestow on them each day the few minutes care that is necessary to keep them in good order, they will do it almost mechanically and not find it a burden as they grow older.

BABY'S NAILS

The baby's nails should be cut as soon as they are long enough to require it. If left untrimmed they sometimes inflict scratches on the tender skin of the face. They can be cleansed by holding the hands for a few moments in warm water, pressing the tips of the fingers away from them and wiping them gently with the soft cloth. Some mothers dust them with violet powder to fill the space, and keep particles of dust from getting beneath and discoloring them.

TRIMMING

It is usual to recommend that nails be paired with a sharp knife. This is a difficult process to accomplish neatly and a pair of curved scissors answer the purpose equally well and are much easier to use.

The outline of a nail should follow the shape of the fingertip and be cut quite close to it. Pointed nails do not look ill on tapered fingers, but when the finger is broad and thick they are out of place.

Toenails should not be cut too short, being long enough at the sides to make them almost square across the top. The mother should pay especial attention to this important point, as it may save much suffering from an ingrowing nail.

CLEANSING

If dirt has accumulated underneath the nails the fingers should be well soaked in warm water, with a little borax or ammonia added to it, to soften and remove it as much as possible. A wooden toothpick is a good instrument to use for this purpose. Ivory or steel, is used roughly or too constantly, wear a ridge on the underside of the nail from which it is difficult to dislodge foreign matter.

Oiling

A few drops of olive oil applied once a week helps to keep the nails pliable and to soften the skin surrounding them so that it can be easily manipulated away from the nail.

Polishing

A polisher or oval piece of wood covered with chamois skin can be purchased at very small cost, and its vigorous use for a few seconds every day makes the nail smooth and glistening and at the same time pushes the surrounding skin into its proper place.

Developing the Lunela

The lunette, lunela, or half-moon-shaped white portion of the nail, really a part of the root, is considered of great beauty when perfectly developed. The skin that the lower part of the nail must be pressed away from it with the point of a polisher and, if it is too abundant or forms the hard ridge, skillfully paired with the sharp knife.

Hangnail

This term is derived from a Saxon word *ange*, meaning troublesome. No one who has suffered from it will doubt the propriety of the derivation. It is a partly detached piece of skin at the root of the nail, inflamed by friction against the hard substance beside it. It should be cut as close to the flesh as possible with the pair of sharp scissors. If there is much inflammation, the finger can be wrapped in a cloth kept wet with a saturated solution of boric acid. When the chief discomfort comes from soreness, it can be anointed with carbolized Vaseline or wet with tincture of witch hazel.

A succession of hang nails shows that the child's general health requires building up.

Ingrowing Nail

This usually occurs on the foot, owing to the pressure of the shoe forcing the nail against the flesh. If the nails are properly cut, that is, nearly square across the top, this accident is very unlikely to happen.

When it is observed, the nail should be scraped with a piece of glass to render it thinner and more pliable. Then, if possible, the point must be gently lifted and the small wedge of cotton wool inserted under it to prevent its bearing itself in the flesh.

When the toe is very much inflamed, it can be kept wrapped in a saturated solution of boracic acid until the condition is a little improved. If the point of the nail is already embedded in the soft part beside it, a surgical operation will be necessary. Sometimes both points are involved, when it is said to be a double ingrowing nail.

SPLINTERS UNDER THE NAIL

If enough of the splinter projects beyond the nail, it can be firmly grasped with a pair of tweezers and drawn out.

If not, a V-shaped piece must be cut from the nail over it with a sharp pointed scissors, when it can be reached with a needle or the tweezers and extracted.

Wrap the finger in linen spread with carbolized Vaseline until it heals.

BITING THE NAILS

In older children this habit sometimes proceeds from an irritable condition of the nervous system for which a physician should prescribe proper remedies. Unstimulating food, as milk, bread, fish and cereals, should be given for a time, meat and eggs being avoided.

Touching the nails with bitter aloes or soaking them in infusion of quassia or covering them with a paste of gum arabic and red pepper, may prevent their being put in the mouth.

When the child is old enough to respond, and appeal to his pride or his affections, or the offer of some substantial reward may effect a cure.

Young children can be made to wear gloves or mittens, or the hands can be kept in bags for a time until the inconvenience leaves the child to wish to cure himself. Not much can be done with older children until the will is enlisted on the side of right.

SUCKING OF FINGERS

Nothing more effectually spoils the shape of the nails and the fingertips then sucking them. This bad habit presses the upper teeth out of place and injures the lower lip.

When the tendency to put the fingers or thumb in the mouth is perceived in a baby, the sleeve should be pinned to the dress or the pillow so the hand cannot be raised in the mouth.

If the habit is established, the means recommended for preventing the nails from being bitten may be tried.

Elizabeth Robinson Scovil *The Care of Children*

It is such a comfort to a baby to suck the thumb it seems a shame to put a stop to such an apparently innocent pleasure. It saves much future annoyance and disfigurement if the child is not allowed to form the habit, and present comfort must be sacrificed to future good.

CARE OF THE FEET
CHAPTER XVIII

RESTING ON THE FEET

The bones of children are very soft and easily bent. They contain a larger proportion of animal matter than the bones of grown persons, in which mineral substances predominate. This peculiarity renders the bones of infants as especially liable to distortion, any undue weight or pressure upon them bends them out of shape.

An active baby should not be allowed to rest its weight on its feet for more than a few seconds at a time. This precaution is particularly necessary if the child is unusually large and heavy. After it is six months old it will begin to feel its feet, resting partially upon them while supported by the mother's hands under its arms.

Creeping is usually the next advance in locomotion, although some babies miss this stage altogether and struggle to their feet, standing alone by the time they are ten months old.

It is a mistake to hold the baby too constantly in the arms. If put down on a rug or blanket on the floor it has a good opportunity to develop the powers of motion and also learns to amuse itself.

WALKING

Proper shoes are a great help in the first efforts to walk. As already mentioned, the soles should be flat, not rounded, and, if the ankles are inclined to be weak, boots that support them for the time being are desirable. Weak ankles should be frequently bathed in salt and water and well rubbed several times a day.

A healthy child shows a desire to pull himself up by some solid article of furniture when he is ready to walk; usually at from ten to fifteen months old.

He should not be forced in any way to anticipate this time by injudicious urging.

If a child does not walk when he is two years old there must be some physical disability which should be investigated.

BATHING

The feet should be bathed in cool water every morning or evening, and well rubbed to bring about the reaction. This keeps the pores open and materially lessens the tendency to take cold.

Elizabeth Robinson Scovil *The Care of Children*

Protecting the Feet

It cannot be too often repeated that the feet are two of the most vulnerable points in the body. Being at a distance from the heart the circulation is often interfered with and cold feet is the result. Warm stocking in cold weather, well-fitting but not too tight shoes, and overshoes for wet days, are absolutely essential to health.

Damp Feet

If the feet are wet the shoes and the stocking should be removed as soon as possible and the feet rubbed with alcohol or spirits of camphor, dry foot-gear being put on, of course.

Children should be instructed not to sit in school with damp feet. If long rubber boots are worn, this accident cannot happen while the boots are whole, unless in the case of some boys to whom length of leg only means a challenge to wade over the top of it.

The feet are sometimes found cold and damp at night and should always be warmed and rubbed before the child goes to sleep.

Excessive Perspiration

This is a most annoying affection, as it usually is accompanied by a disagreeable odor. Special attention should be paid to cleanliness and the following liniment may be used:

Tannic acid, two drams, or teaspoonfuls. Alcohol, eight ounces, or sixteen tablespoonfuls. This preparation stains clothing.

It may be applied twice a day. After it is dry dust the feet with finely powdered French chalk. Do not use the vegetable powder, as cornstarch, for this is unfavorably affected by the heat and moisture.

The stockings should be changed frequently.

Corns

Corns are nature's effort to protect the soft tissues of the foot by forming a callus to sustain the pressure.

They are evidences of the faulty construction of shoes, and in some cases of the vanity that persists in wearing shoes too small for the foot.

With children in a shoe that has caused the mischief should be abandoned.

If there is much tenderness a section of lemon can be bound over the sore spot at night. When the corn is between the toes a wad of cotton wool gives great relief. If outside the toe a circle of felt with a hole in the middle can be placed over it, and secured with sticking plaster.

After soaking the foot in warm water the horny substance of the corn can be pared away, and if there is subsequent relief from the pressure, it will probably be cured without further trouble.

A bunion is an enlargement and inflammation of the joint of a toe, usually of the great toe. It is not very common in children. Removal of pressure and painting the part with tincture of iodine will often be effectual if it is discovered early. Later, when there is much inflammation, and perhaps matter has formed, it should be seen by a physician.

CHAFED HEEL

Children often suffer much from the heel having been rubbed by a badly-fitting shoe, or one that has a rough projection, where the seam is at the back of the uppers. A circular piece of rubber plaster, applied when the pain is first complained of, will give complete relief. If the skin is rubbed off, the place must be dressed with a little cold cream over the night and the plaster applied over fresh dressing in the morning.

Ingrowing nails have already been mentioned.

CHILBLAINS

Chilblains are painfully red inflamed spots on the toes, heels, and sometimes on the fingers, occasioned by exposure to cold. On their first appearance, they may be painted with iodine, or rubbed with an ointment of one part of ground mustard mixed with three parts of lard. Camphorated oil sometimes gives relief. If neglected, they may ulcerate and should then be dressed with balsam of Peru spread on linen and washed every day with a weak solution of carbolic acid.

The following ointment is said to prevent the occurrence of this condition:

Oxide of zinc, one and a half ounces;
Glycerin, one and a half ounces;
Lanolin, one and a half ounces.

It should be well rubbed in after washing.

Elizabeth Robinson Scovil *The Care of Children*

AILMENTS
CHAPTER XIX

SIMPLE REMEDIES

It cannot be too earnestly impressed upon the mother that children need very little medicine, and that only the simplest remedy should be given to them without the advice of a doctor.

Many of their ailments arise from a disordered digestion. A gentle laxative will often carry off the offending substance, and a small dose of Castor oil, citrate of magnesia, Rochelle salts, or spice syrup of rhubarb may be ventured on with perfect safety. Compound and licorice powder is the safe laxative. It owes its efficacy to the Sina it contains. Half a teaspoon may be given to a child of four years old at bedtime, and the dose increase to a teaspoonful for older children. It is easily taken mixed with a little water, as the taste is not especially disagreeable.

More powerful remedies may do more harm than good when administered by the inexperienced. Attention to the diet, perfect cleanliness, good ventilation, and sufficient sleep are more valuable as curative measures than most of the drugs in the pharmacopeia.

FEVERISHNESS

A child's temperature rises very easily, and an elevation does not mean as much as in an adult.

A clinical thermometer is a useful instrument for the mother to have. The normal temperature is 98.4°F.

If a child is flushed and hot at night, a warm bath should be given, and the saline laxative, as the teaspoonful of Rochelle salts, or more according to age. Cold water is always admissible, but it is better not to have it iced. Lumps of ice may be given, as they dissolve slowly, and do not precipitate a quantity of ice-cold fluid into the stomach at once. Ice, however, rather increases than the assuages thirst.

Local symptoms, as sore throat, pain in the chest, etc., may be treated by the proper applications. If the child is suffering, and seems very ill, the doctor should be sent for. If not, it is safe to wait until the morning when, if there is no improvement, he certainly should be summoned. Often in the evening temperature of over 103°F will have some subsided in twelve hours, leaving apparently no ill effects.

Colic

The symptoms are severe pain in the abdomen, which is generally relieved by pressure, as lying on the stomach. There is no fever, and the attack can often be traced to an indigestible article of food, as green apples, or too large a quantity of nuts.

Heat can be applied to the seat of pain by means of the invaluable rubber hot water bag, which is indispensable in every household. Hot drinks can be given, as essence of peppermint, or half a teaspoonful of tincture of ginger in hot water.

If the attack is very severe, an enema of hot water will help to give relief. A dose of castor oil should be given at night.

If nuts have been partaken of too freely, a teaspoonful of salt dissolved in hot water is the best remedy.

The diet should be regulated after the attack to prevent its recurrence.

In young babies, colic is usually the result of overfeeding or indigestion. Yet sometimes the utmost attention to diet seems powerless to avert it.

The pain arises from the distension of the stomach and intestines by an accumulation of gas or "wind", arising from the fermentation of the food.

When a baby cries from colic, the knees are drawn up, the abdomen feels hard and tense, the hands and feet are cold and relief follows an expulsion of gas.

Regulation of the quantity and quality of the food is important. Warmth and friction help to cut short an attack.

The pain comes on with some babies at a certain time every day. When this is the case, the enemy can sometimes be circumvented by wrapping the baby in a blanket with a hot-water bag before the hour when the attack may be expected.

Rubbing the bowels with the warm hand, beginning the low down on the right side, bringing the hand up, across the abdomen and down the left side, may give relief. The feet should be warmly wrapped in flannel and kept in a hot-water bag.

A few teaspoonfuls of warm lime water may be given or two or three drops of essence of peppermint in hot water — not sweetened — as sugar tends to aggravate the fermentation. Plain warm water may be used.

In severe cases an enema of warm water given with an infant's rectal syringe may bring relief. A hot bath can be tried when other means fail.

Elizabeth Robinson Scovil *The Care of Children*

CRYING

Babies cry from other causes than colic and it is well to bear these in mind. They do occasionally have an opportunity to cry from hunger, as when a longer sleep than usual has lengthened the interval between two meals or when the last meal has from any cause been a small one. This cry is stilled after food, while that from colic is increased by feeding. A baby sometimes cries from thirst as well as hunger and one or two spoonfuls of water may be a panacea.

If the water is not passed at proper intervals, it causes discomfort. The legs are drawn up to lessen the pressure and the child frets and wails. Flannels rung out of very hot water and laid over the lower part of the abdomen may relieve this condition. The heat and moisture cause relaxation and the water escapes.

When a rash is present the possibility of irritation from this source should be remembered. It can be bathed with a solution of baking soda in water.

Unguarded pins are not put into the clothes of the modern baby and, as no tight bands confine it, these causes of tears are eliminated.

A cry is the natural expression of discomfort from any cause. A baby does not shed tears until it is nearly three months old, as they are not secreted before that time.

CONSTIPATION

This is one of the most common ailments of childhood and may be relieved in a variety of ways.

With older children attention to the diet is often all that is necessary to give relief and this means has already been touched upon.

Massage, or careful rubbing and kneading of the abdomen, either with warm oil or without, will often produce a movement.

When the intestine is inactive, they can be induced to move by a suppository.

The simplest for a young baby is a piece of white writing paper twisted into a cone about four inches long. The end is oiled and gently passed into the rectum for about an inch.

A suppository can be made by scraping a piece of white soap to the thickness of a lead pencil and inserting about two inches. It is of course expelled with the movement.

Molasses boiled to the consistency of candy and shaped into suppositories is very effectual.

Prunes covered with water, boiled until they form a pulp and then strained, make an excellent laxative. A teaspoonful of the water can be given every morning to a baby six months old, increasing the dose for older ones.

Half a teaspoonful of flake mana can be added to the milk once a day and repeated, if necessary.

It is unwise to give castor oil constantly, or any of the patent cathartic medicines, as they only give temporary relief and increase the difficulty ultimately.

When it is necessary to effective movement in obstinate constipation, an enema of one ounce, or two tablespoonfuls, of warm oil can be given; or a larger quantity of warm soap suds.

It is very important to establish regular habits. A baby can be held out at the same hour every morning and evening after it is a month old. Some children seldom soil the napkin after the first six weeks.

Other children should be required to make an effort to have a movement every morning, but ineffectual straining should not be permitted, as there is danger of the lower part of the bowel prolapsing or coming down.

The discharge should be soft, yet formed, except in babies under two years old. If it is in hard, round balls, it has been retrained retained for some time and more fluid is needed and should be given. There are children who do not seem to be able to have a movement oftener than every other day. If the general health is good this is not a ground for anxiety.

DIARRHEA

During the first few weeks of a baby's life there are usually three or four movements during the twenty-four hours. These gradually decrease in number until, when the child is two years old, eating a variety of solid food, there is only one a day.

While the diet is principally milk, the motions will be yellow in color and soft is inconsistency. If white curds of milk appear in them the food is not being properly digested. It may be lessened in quantity for a time and a little more lime water added to it.

When the movements are clay-colored the liver is torpid and the doctor should be consulted.

If a child is taking iron or bismuth, the excretion will be very dark, almost black. Should there be a stricture of the bowel, the matter will be small in size, sometimes not larger than a pipe stem.

When the movements increase in frequency beyond the normal limit and become greenish in color and watery and consistency, we say the child has diarrhea.

This is an evidence of some disturbance of the intestinal tract, usually from indigestion.

If it has been preceded by constipation, a dose of castor oil will probably give relief, removing the offending substance. To a young baby, three or four drops

Elizabeth Robinson Scovil *The Care of Children*

may be given every three hours for four or five doses, or until there has been a free evacuation.

For a child six months old, a teaspoonful once will be sufficient. The dose can be increased to a tablespoonful for a child of six years. Children bear castor oil well.

The food should always be attended to when diarrhea is present.

If the evacuations become white and watery, containing mucus and, perhaps, streaks of blood, with the constant straining and desire to have a movement the disease is known as dysentery. The inflammation has extended to the large intestine.

Diarrhea should not be allowed to go on long and unchecked. The physician should be consulted if home remedies are ineffectual.

For older children rest in bed and restricted diet will often effect a cure. A flannel bandage should be worn during the day and night, as warmth over the bowels is important.

Hiccough

Hiccough, or hiccup, is usually a symptom of little importance. It is caused by a spasmodic contraction of the diaphragm, the muscle separating the chest from the abdomen. It may arise from the presence of too much food, wind, or gas, in the stomach. Often diverting the child's mind is all that is necessary. A sudden, quick movement of a baby, or patting it on the back, telling an older child to hold his breath while he counts twenty slowly, is sometimes effectual. In obstinate cases, two drops of spirits of camphor on sugar may be given to a child of three years old, and increased to ten for one of fifteen.

COLDS
Prevention

In northern climates the cold is one of the most common ills of childhood. There is a great difference in the susceptibility of children, some taking cold much more easily than others. It attacks special points, as the head or the chest, and when one is found to be vulnerable it must be specially guarded.

Sponging with cool salt and water and accustoming the child to live in a well-ventilated room at not too high a temperature, helps to ensure immunity.

If the chest is liable to be attacked it is well to rub it with warm oil, both back and front, at night, and keep a fold of cotton batting, or wadding, over it during the day.

Cold in the Head

A variety of cold in the head called snuffles, sometimes observed in a young baby, should always be reported to the doctor, as it may indicate constitutional disease.

When the nose is obstructed, rubbing it with Vaseline or warm oil will sometimes give relief, carrying it inside with a camel's-hair brush. Older children may inhale cologne with the drop of ammonia water in it. Spirits of camphor may be used in the same way. Gently syringing nostrils with warm salt and water is said to be an effectual remedy. A small glass syringe with a blunt nose is the best for this purpose.

Hoarseness

This is caused by inflammation of the larynx, the enlargement at the top of the windpipe that contains the vocal cords. A warm poultice or flannels rung out of hot water are sometimes useful. The throat should be covered with dry flannel the next day. Inhaling the steam from a pitcher of boiling water helps to relax the tension. Thirty drops of compound tincture of benzoin can be added to the water. A few drops of lemon juice given on sugar and repeated frequently is a pleasant remedy.

Cold in the Chest

This is known to physicians as bronchitis, or inflammation of the bronchial tubes. The child is feverish, with some cough and a feeling of tightness in the chest and throat perhaps a dull pain. The feet should be soaked in hot water with a little mustard added to it and a warm poultice applied to the chest. This must be changed every hour to keep up the heat. When a poultice cannot be obtained, the chest can be rubbed with warm camphorated oil and covered with flannel. A warm drink — flaxseed tea flavored with lemon juice is good — can be given at bedtime. If the cough is tight, ten to twenty drops of wine of ipecac can be given to a child two years old.

It is especially important that children with delicate chests should wear flannel and have the feet protected with woolen stockings.

When wool next to the skin is unbearably irritating, as is undoubtedly is to some hypersensitive children, very thin cotton stockings can be worn underneath the others and gauze shirts and drawers inside the woolen ones.

There is no more effectual measure for the prevention of colds than thoroughly protecting the extremities, particularly the feet. Overshoes should be worn in wet walking and removed on entering the house. If the shoes are damp, the evaporation as they dry carries off the heat from the feet, rendering them cold

Elizabeth Robinson Scovil *The Care of Children*

and damp, and almost certainly brings on the symptoms of a cold.

If a child's feet are habitually cold, the cause should be sought for and removed.

Warmer foot coverings must be provided, and the circulation stimulated by brisk rubbing night and morning.

Snoring

Children as well as grown up persons should keep the mouth shut and breathe through the nostrils.

Snoring is a danger signal, showing that something is wrong with the throat or the nasal passages, presenting an impediment to proper breathing.

The tonsils, or the little glands on each side of the throat at the back of the tongue, may be enlarged, partially filling up the passage from the throat to the nose, preventing the free access of air in that way. If they are much inflamed, the child should be taken to a surgeon, who will apply some astringent application, or, if necessary, remove the offending glands, not a serious operation usually.

Snoring may proceed from catarrh of the throat or nose. There may be a growth obstructing the nasal passage. Whatever the cause, it should be found and treated, as persistent breathing through the mouth impairs the capacity of the chest, injures the lungs and opens the way the many ills difficult, if not impossible, to cure in after years.

SORE MOUTH
Thrush

Young babies and even older children sometimes have tiny white patches in the mouth, which are really a fungoid growth like little toadstools. They look like specks of milk. Sometimes they extend through the whole digestive tract, causing the movements to become greenish, and upsetting the digestion.

It is usually caused by want of cleanliness. The nursing bottle, or nipple, may be neglected; the mouth may not have been swabbed faithfully after food was given, or the diet may be improper, causing disturbance of the stomach. Remove every exciting outside cause by exquisite cleanliness of bottle, nipple, and mouth. Use a saturated solution of boracic acid, instead of clear water, to swab the mouth, and if the patches appear at the anus, or opening of the bowel, sprinkle them with a powder made of equal parts of boracic acid, oxide of zinc, and French chalk.

A saturated solution is made by dissolving in the water all the boracic acid it will take up, as is shown by some of the crystals remaining undissolved at the bottom of the bottle. Boracic acid can be obtained from the apothecary in small crystals and can be powdered.

With older children, the little canker sores that sometimes come inside the mouth, at the junction of the lips with the jaws, can be cured by dusting them with powdered alum.

COLD SORES

Cold sores appearing at the corners of the lips outside can be touched with spirits of camphor in the early stages, which will probably prevent their farther development. If it is too late for this treatment, Vaseline, or cold cream, is the best application.

CRACKED LIPS

When the lips are roughened and cracked, a mixture of four teaspoonfuls of glycerin and one of the compound tincture of benzoin is an excellent emollient to apply.

GUM BOILS

Gum boils show some inflammation at the root of the tooth and require the attention of a dentist. A tiny square of capsicum plaster over the offending part helps to relieve the condition for the time.

SORE THROAT

This may be a comparatively trifling ailment, or it may be the beginning of a disease that involves a struggle between life and death.

A baby's throat can be examined by holding it towards a window, or a bright light, tipping back the head, pressing down the chin to open the mouth, and holding down the tongue with a flat toothbrush, or spoon handle.

An older child, if amenable to the reason, can be made to show the throat by telling it to open the mouth and say "ah". Some children find it impossible to hold down the tongue voluntarily, and then it must be depressed with a spoon handle. If a child is accustomed to do this occasionally when in health, it will not be so difficult to induce it to repeat the performance when it is really necessary.

The throat is very sensitive in children and responds quickly to any derangement of the system. Cold, impure air, or any digestive disturbance, inflames the delicate membrane that lines it.

In the sore throat resulting from cold the mucous membrane is congested, being a darker red than usual from the presence of an extra quantity of blood. A

Elizabeth Robinson Scovil *The Care of Children*

folded piece of cotton wrung out of cold water with a flannel band laid over it, renewed as it becomes dry, will often be all that is needed to give relief. A gentle laxative, as milk of magnesia, may be given if indigestion is suspected.

Sometimes there is slight tenderness on pressing the outside. The uvula, or pointed palate that hangs at the back of the mouth may be swelled, and there may be a little mucus, but no white spots or patches. There may be a good deal of pain in swallowing, as the food presses on the inflamed surfaces, and only soft things, or liquids, should be given.

There is another form of sore throat in which the tonsils principally are affected. They can be felt a little swelled and hard on the outside of the throat, and inside small spots, or patches, like little ulcers, white or yellow in color, appear on them. These are confined to the tonsils, and do not extend to the uvula, or pointed part of the soft palate, the roof of the mouth, or backwards towards the throat. The spots can be touched with a camel's-hair brush dipped in compound tincture of benzoin, or borax and glycerin, the cold bandage applied, and a mild laxative given. The child should be kept indoors, and in bed if more comfortable there; twenty-four hours will probably show great improvement. If not, send for the doctor, as it is not safe to delay longer, lest it should be a serious case.

STIFF NECK

This affliction frequently occurs in children who have a tendency to rheumatism, and in those who for any reason are not as strong and vigorous as usual. Hot fomentations, that is, flannels wrung out of hot water, can be applied to the neck and frequently removed, and the neck bound in flannel.

The diet should be attended to, being more nutritious than usual. A teaspoonful of Rochelle salts can be given in the morning for two or three days, and if the general condition is feeble, the doctor should be asked to prescribe a tonic.

COUGH

This may be a symptom of whooping cough, or croup, or merely due to a slight irritation of the lining membrane of the windpipe. If it is persistent, or annoying, inhaling the steam from hot water with thirty drops of compound tincture of benzoin mixed with it may allay it, or the application of hot fomentations to the throat. If it is very severe, fifteen drops of wine of ipecac may be given, and repeated twice. Half a teaspoonful of glycerin given in warm milk is soothing. Cough medicine should be avoided, as they disorder the stomach and do little good.

RASHES

These are of many different kinds and proceed from a variety of causes. Sometimes they are infectious, as in scarlet fever, or the affection known as the itch; sometimes confined to the child himself, and meaning no more than a disordered digestion.

ERYTHEMA

Erythema, or heat rash, is red spots varying in size from the head of a hat pin to a five-cent piece. They are slightly hard and itch, coming on the legs, arms, back and shoulders. After a day or two they disappear, and fresh crop comes out. There is a red wing around each one which distinguishes the eruption from chicken pox.

They can be anointed with Vaseline, or cold cream, and a little fluid magnesia, or milk of magnesia given as a laxative. Avoid oatmeal, meat and sugar in the food for at time.

ROSEOLA

This rash is sometimes confounded with measles, or scarlet fever. Unlike these diseases there is no fever, the symptoms of cold in the head, as in measles, and sore throat, as in scarlet fever, are absent.

It requires very little treatment, confinement to the house, a light diet and mild laxative being all that is needed.

URTICARIA

Urticaria, or nettle rash, also known as hives, is an eruption that causes much misery to many children. It appears in the form of large white blotches surrounded with red and itches intensely. Certain articles of food, as strawberries, will provoke an attack in some cases. When these are known they must be avoided. Bathing the spots in a solution of bicarbonate of soda, or water with a few drops of ammonia, gives temporary relief. If it is known to have been caused by the diet, a little castor oil may be given, and if it persists a few spoonfuls of fluid magnesia daily until it disappears.

ECZEMA

There are several forms of this affection of the skin. In the most common the cuticle comes off in dry rashes, leaving cracks from which a fluid exudes. There is usually itching, which is relieved by Vaseline spread on linen and applied. It may last for years and a physician should always be consulted.

Meat, sugar and oatmeal should be avoided in the diet.

Elizabeth Robinson Scovil *The Care of Children*

There are some rashes and other affections of the skin which are hereditary. When either parent is afflicted in this way, the earliest symptoms should be carefully observed and the case placed under the care of a physician.

Mosquito Bites

A wash that will help to relieve the irritation is made as follows:

> Lime water, one pint; oxide of zinc, one teaspoonful; glycerin, one teaspoonful.

When this dries, dust the bites with equal parts of finely powdered boracic acid and starch.

Ring Worm

This is a troublesome disease of the scalp, infectious amongst children. The hair comes off in patches, leaving only the roughened, broken bristles, and each spot is surrounded by an oval or circular border sometimes inflamed, from which it derives its popular name of ring-worm.

Children afflicted with it require stimulating food, meat, broths, eggs, etc., and to be built up by saltwater baths, plenty of fresh air and exercise. A physician should see the case, as iron and some other tonic may be needed. The spots can be touched with tincture of iodine applied with a brush. Various ointments are prescribed, but is it is not safe to use most of them without the advice of a physician.

The disease may be communicated to grown persons; then it attacks other parts of the body and not the head. In spite of the name it is not caused by a worm, but, as some authorities claim, by a tiny fungus plant, or, as others say, simply by a degeneration of the cells of the skin and hair. It is never said to cause baldness. The natural tendency is towards a cure, though it may last for several years if it is not properly treated.

Itch

School children often contract this disagreeable affection. The technical name is scabies, and it is also known as Scotch fiddle. It is caused by the presence of a parasite which burrows under the skin between the fingers, on the inside of the wrists and elbows and sometimes on the abdomen and legs.

The trace left by the parasites looks like an old pin scratch, and as the irritation is great the victim's own nails soon add to it.

Sulphur ointment is the application generally used. It should be freely applied and well rubbed in, particularly at night, and followed by a warm bath in the morning.

The use of the ointment may be continued for a week or ten days, and then benzoated lard should be submitted. The sulfur irritates the skin and keeps up the inflammation if its use is prolonged.

When the hands are affected gloves should be worn to prevent the infection of others.

WORMS

The only positive proof of the presence of worms in the intestine is their appearance in the motions. Vermifuges should not be given without this proof, and more harm may be done than good.

There are two varieties: the tiny pin worms, looking like white threads, and round worms, which resemble the common earthworm in appearance, and are several inches in length.

When a child has shooting pains in the abdomen, nausea and vomiting without apparent cause, fetid breath, itching nose, or of the anus, the lower opening of the bowel, the movements should be carefully examined.

If thread worms are detected a handful of quassia chips should be put to soak in a quart of water. After eight to ten hours the water is strained off and about half a pint, slightly warmed, administered as an enema with an ordinary bulb syringe. This will be retained for some time and can be followed in an hour with an enema of plain warm water.

A teaspoonful of Rochelle salts can be given at night and repeated as necessary.

The greatest cleanliness must be observed, the anus being frequently washed with warm soap and water, the nails kept short, washed and cleansed often, that the parasites may not lodge beneath them and carried to other parts.

Round worms will not easily escape when they appear in the motions.

Santonin is the remedy most highly recommended, but as it is a powerful medicine, producing convulsions in overdose, and has proved fatal, it cannot be given without a physician's prescription. It is followed by a dose of castor oil. It can be obtained in tablets made up with chocolate, a pleasant way of administering it.

BED WETTING

This is very common among children, especially boys. Scolding and punishing are not of the slightest use. It is due to an abnormal condition which must have proper treatment for its relief.

Elizabeth Robinson Scovil *The Care of Children*

It is well to protect the bed with a piece of rubber sheeting a yard wide and long enough to tuck firmly under the mattress on each side. Over this firmly under the mattress on each side. Over this can be laid a pad made of several thicknesses of newspaper, with a layer of cotton waste on top, covered with a piece of old cotton. This can be rolled up and burned in the morning.

If the mother recognizes that the occurrence is a misfortune and not a fault, and prepares for it, she will find it much more easy to bear.

Proper medicine is required for its cure and this only a doctor can prescribe.

The child should be taken up the last thing before the mother goes to bed, and once or twice in the night. Sometimes raising the foot of the bed four to five inches is effectual in preventing the accident. Lying on the side renders it less likely to happen, and it used to be the practice to tie an empty spool by a string round the waist so that when the little sleeper turned on his back the pressure would waken him.

Night Terror

A child will sometimes waken from sleep with a scream of terror, having apparently had a distressing dream which has terrified him beyond measure.

These attacks answer to the nightmare that afflicts his elders and can generally be traced to some imprudence of diet or to constipation.

A teaspoonful of spiced syrup of rhubarb, or any gentle laxative, will remove the cause and care must be taken that the indigestible article of food that produced the symptoms is not given again. The last meal of the day should be very simple, as bread and milk.

The mother should make sure that the child is not being told alarming stories nor frightened in any way by the nurse or other servants.

If the attacks continue a physician should be consulted.

Sleeplessness

Children of a restless, nervous temperament sometimes feel great difficulty in going to sleep. It is not willful naughtiness that prevents the poor little thing from shutting their eyes and lysing still as they are ordered to do. It is simply a physical inability to compose themselves to sleep.

Such children should have a warm bath at bedtime, followed by gentle friction to the whole body. A cup of warm milk is an excellent hypnotic for old or young. If the feet are cold they should be chafed and placed on a hot-water bag. An ice bag or a cloth wrung out of ice water can be applied to the back of the neck at the same time.

The presence of too much blood in the brain renders natural sleep impossible and the object is to draw away as much blood as possible.

Excitable children should not be told stories or read to at bedtime not allowed to romp while undressing. Darkness is especially soothing to the tired nerves and, unless the child has a nervous terror of it, the light should never be left burning.

GROWING PAINS

Delicate children of a nervous temperament often suffer from intense pain in the legs and knee-joint, familiarly known as growing pains. They are apt to come on at night, after the fatigue of the day. Warmth and friction is the best treatment. The legs can be thoroughly rubbed with spirits of camphor or any simply stimulating liniment, wrapped in flannel and a hot-water bag applied to them.

A warm drink will aid the soothing process. A warm bath, 98°F, containing two ounces, about two tablespoonfuls, of carbonate of soda, common washing soda, at each three gallons of water is recommended. It should be given at night.

A fixed pain on the inside of the knee should not be disregarded, as it may point to disease of the hip.

BOILS

These occur most often in children from eight to ten years old, particularly in boys. They are apt to come where there is friction or pressure from the clothing, though sometimes they appear on the face. They are often preceded by itching and it is said that if at this stage the tiny hair on the surface is pulled out, the formation will be prevented. An almost unfailing remedy, although a severe one for the moment, is to dip a match, the end covered with phosphorous being first taken off, into pure carbolic acid and to touch the pimple directly in the middle. It acts like fire, cauterizing the part and stops the progress of the boil.

When a head has formed, surrounded with a hard inflamed surface, it must be poulticed with a flaxseed poultice until the induration is softened and the boil discharges, and then dressed with Vaseline or any soothing ointment,

It is said that the development of boils is due to dryness of the skin and if the part is faithfully rubbed with thick cream, fresh butter or any fatty substance, they may be prevented.

In children boils show a depressed state of the system. Nutritious food should be given and tonics may be required.

Elizabeth Robinson Scovil *The Care of Children*

Chafing

It is sometimes difficult to prevent chafing in babies with delicate skin. The great preventative is keeping them dry and well powdered in the creases where surfaces touch one another. Sometimes, older children suffer from it if they are very fat or perspire freely. French chalk makes an inexpensive and efficient powder, it can be scented with powdered orris root if desired.

If the skin is much reddened it is well to use sub-nitrate of bismuth. The parts should be washed in thin, boiled starch instead of plain water and as seldom as possible. In powdering, shake the powder on from the puff, do not touch the abraded surface more than is absolutely necessary.

Chapped Hands

In winter the hands often become rough, and are said to be chapped. Some skins crack and bleed, so that much discomfort is produced. The following is an excellent wash: Glycerin, three teaspoonfuls; rose water, four tablespoonfuls; compound tincture of benzoin, half a teaspoonful. It should be put on after washing the hands, and always at night. The skin heals more rapidly if gloves are worn at night. When the hands are washed they should be dried by patting with a soft towel, rubbing being avoided.

Inflammation of the Breasts

The breasts of a young baby may swell and a milk-like fluid ooze from them. This should not be pressed out nor the breasts manipulated in any way. If they are very hard, red, and seem tender when touched a flannel wrung out of hot water can be laid over them, and renewed every ten minutes as it grows cool, until the application has continued an hour or more. Cover the flannel with a strip of oiled silk, or India-rubber cloth, to retain the heat.

The treatment can be repeated until the condition is relieved.

Headache

Young children are not apt to have headache from slight disturbance of the digestion, or over-strain, as adults are. When this symptom is present in them, it indicates some more serious affection, and the cause should be diligently sought for.

In older children headache frequently results from sitting in a badly ventilated school-room, from constipation, or want of attention to some of the laws of health.

Delicate, nervous children frequently bring it on by over-study. This may not be because they have too many lessons for a vigorous child, but that the brain is taxed beyond their physical powers. The remedy is to lessen the amount of brain work until the body can be brought into a condition to responds to the call made upon it. A thoroughly healthy child seldom over-studies.

Late hours are a frequent cause of headache amongst young people. They do not have sufficient sleep to rest the brain and nerves.

The tendency to sick headache is sometimes inherited. When this is not the case the cause may be found in bad ventilation, when the vitiated air acts as poison to the system, in over-study, in a debilitated state of the system, requiring tonics and a generous diet, or in the disturbance attending the cutting of the second teeth.

A common cause of headache in children is eyestrain. The forehead and front of the head is especially affected. It follows prolonged use of the eyes, as at school, and can be relieved by proper glasses.

There may be violent headache after an attack of coughing in whooping cough. Intense headache may indicate disease of the brain, when there is usually a shrinking from light.

In young babies, restlessly moving the head from side to side on the pillow indicates pain in the head or ear, and may be one of the early symptoms of rickets.

When headache persists a physician should be consulted. He may be able to discover the cause and give advice, which if faithfully followed will result in a permanent cure.

CATARRH

Catarrh is a discharge of fluid from the mucous membrane, usually of the nasal passages; at least that is the form which the mother most often first perceives. It generally results from cold, becoming chronic after repeated colds in the head.

The child may sneeze constantly, breathes through the nose with difficulty, often complains of headache or earache, and expectorates frequently.

Home treatment cannot be depended upon for the cure of catarrh; it often taxes the skill of the physician. Various means are employed, as syringing the nose with different fluid, always warm, spraying it with heated Vaseline or glycerin, and much patience is needed to continue the applications until it is relieved.

THE MEDICINE BOX

The mother will find it convenient to have in a box, or a safe corner of the closet shelf, a few simple remedies to use in time of need.

It is best only to have a small quantity of any drug and renew it as it is

Elizabeth Robinson Scovil *The Care of Children*

required. Oils especially do hot keep well, and castor oil should be watched lest it become rancid. The following will be found useful:

> Compound liquorice powder,
> Spiced syrup of rhubarb,
> Castor oil,
> Citrate of magnesia,
> Wine of ipecac,
> Powdered alum,
> Tincture of ginger,
> Essence of peppermint,
> Soda mint tablets.

One of the first four laxatives will usually give relief in any ordinary case. The wine of ipecac and alum are efficient emetics. The ginger, or peppermint will relieve pain in the stomach, and the soda mint checks nausea and relieves flatulence.

How To Give Medicine

Prepare it so it may be as little disagreeable as possible.

Oils

Castor oil may be stirred into warm milk, flavored with a few drops of essence of peppermint and a little sugar added. If taken through a glass tube, it is less distasteful.

It may be carefully poured into a wineglass of ice water and a small piece of ice held in the ought before taking it. The cold benumbs the nerves of taste and the ball which the oil forms in the ice water glides down very easily. A little lemon juice on sugar will remove any flavor that may remain.

Cod-liver oil can be made into an emulsion with the yolk of an egg, beating it like mayonnaise, adding a few drops of oil at the time; flavor with extract of bitter almond or lemon, and sweeten if desired. A little salt taken after the pure oil removes the traces of it, and baked apple is efficacious for the same purpose.

Powders

Mix them with syrup or conceal them in a dessert spoonful of jam, or a split fig. Tasteless ones can be given dry on the tongue, followed by a draught of water. Small ones may be sprinkled on a spoonful of chipped ice.

PILLS

It is often difficult to swallow a small pill. The muscles of the throat cannot grasp it firmly to push it down because of its want of bulk. It can be put into jam or pressed into a square of bread cut like dice.

TABLETS

Tablets, which are so often prescribed now, can be treated like pills or dissolved in a spoonful of water.

Medicine that has a disagreeable odor should not be held under the nose.

A little cologne on a handkerchief to sniff will divert the child's attention.

In giving a nauseous drug that has to be dissolved, put it in as little water as possible and follow it with as much as will be taken.

When liquids are given the spoon should be put well into the mouth, tipped and withdrawn quickly, as the child cannot swallow while the tongue is held down.

Do not destroy confidence in the truthfulness of grown persons by saying the medicine is not nasty. Say nothing about it, or make a virtue of the bravery of taking it when it is not nice.

Elizabeth Robinson Scovil *The Care of Children*

PHYSICAL DEFORMITIES
CHAPTER XX

BOW LEGS

This deformity is always a source of anxiety to mothers. It is apt to occur in children who are suffering from rickets. Much may be done to correct it by persistent pressing and rubbing of the limb in the opposite direction from the curve. Children's bones are so much softer than those of grown persons that they are affected by pressure as an adults could not be. Bathing with salt and water is beneficial as a tonic; and attention to the food and general health is indispensable.

If the child is old enough to walk, a pair of shoes should be chosen without heels, and a layer or two of thick leather nailed the entire length of the soles on the outer sides. This should be shaved thin towards the middle of the sole not to make an uncomfortable ridge under the foot.

KNOCK KNEES

In this affection the knees touch and the feet are turned in. It also occurs in rickets, though it may arise from other causes. The same general treatment can be pursued as in bowlegs. In this case the shoes must have the leather nailed on the inner side of the sole, turning the foot out and keeping the knees apart.

This simple device has proved effective when a cumbersome and expensive apparatus could not be worn on account of its weight.

FLAT FOOT

In this condition that arch of the foot is flattened. In standing, instead of the natural curve of the inner side being well defined, the whole side of the foot touches the ground.

When the arch has given way from overstrain, the muscles being too weak to support the weight they had to bear, there is always pain.

Many persons suffer great inconvenience for years without the true cause being recognized.

Great relief can be given by proper cushions, or pads, placed under the sole. A surgeon should be consulted and his advice followed.

Club Foot

This deformity is so well marked that it cannot escape notice. The child should have the advantage of professional skill as early as possible. Some cases can be much benefited by proper bandages, skillfully applied, or other mechanical means; in others an operation is the only hope of correcting the disfigurement.

Dr. Bradford says that in an infant a spasm of the muscles, turning the foot inwards, has been mistaken for a case of true club foot. This is temporary, passing away in a short time.

Hip Disease

This is a chronic affection of the hip joint arising from various causes. It is common in delicate children and may be brought on by a fall, or a blow, that would produce no serious result in a healthy child.

The first symptom is lameness, which is observed before there is any pain. The child limps in the morning and the stiffness seems to wear off as the day advances and the leg is more used. Sometimes there is a good deal of pain in the knee, or the thigh above the knee; in other cases there is for a time little complaint of pain.

If the leg cannot be brought upwards on the abdomen without pain, when a child is lying on his back, disease of the hip joint may be feared.

The parts must be kept absolutely still. In order to accomplish this, suitable splints or a proper apparatus must be applied by a surgeon and the child kept in bed.

This relieves the pain and is the most speedy way to recovery. The room must be well-ventilated, plenty of sunshine admitted, and the food be nourishing and easily digested.

Curvature of the Spine

While a mother should not be nervously over-anxious about the health and development of her children, she should be on the watch to detect as soon as possible any deviation from the normal condition. Defects in symmetry especially can be more easily remedied while the child is young and no neglect of observation should permit them to become fixed without at least an effort having been made to relieve them.

When a child is having his bath is a good time to examine him carefully. If the spine is not found perfectly straight, particularly if deflection exists between or near the shoulders, a surgeon should be informed of it. Sometimes the child holds one shoulder higher than the other, or one shoulder-blade projects more

Elizabeth Robinson Scovil *The Care of Children*

than its fellow. If the two sides of the body are not alike in every respect, suspicion should be excited.

PIGEON BREAST

Sometimes the ribs in front are flattened and the breast bone projects unduly, forming what is known as pigeon breasts.

Very much can be done for the relief and cure of deformity of the spine by means of proper physical exercises, carried out under the direction of the surgeon.

These consist of improving the capacity of the chest by deep inhalations of air, movements of the head, arms and body, and exercises with dumbbells.

Sometimes a plaster jacket or steel brace is needed.

The treatment must be faithfully kept up for many months; no very rapid improvement can be expected, but, unless there is disease of the bone, the outlook is favorable.

HARE LIP

In this deformity the upper lip is divided, sometimes in the middle and sometimes in two places.

Children are born with it and it may also occur from accident, as falling on a sharp stone.

In a young baby it is usually considered best to operate upon it early. The surgeon pares the sides of the cleft, brings the edges together and secures the with stitches or pins with sutures twisted across them.

Wounds of the face heal very quickly; in a short time the edges grow together, if the operation is successful, and only a scar remains to show where the opening was.

The great difficulty in the nursing is to prevent the child from crying, as any strain on the parts tends to draw them apart. He must be fed with a spoon, as the attempt to suck would have the same result.

The deformity is said to be more common with boys than girls and takes its name from its resemblance to the cleft upper lip of the hare.

CLEFT PALATE

The fissure of the lip may extend through the gum, across the hard palate, or roof of the mouth, and the soft palate behind it. There are also cases of cleft palate without the hare lip.

The child cannot suck and when fed with a spoon the liquid is apt to be forced upwards into the opening of the nasal passage within the mouth.

A rubber nipple has been invented with a flap of rubber attached to it, which is pressed against the roof of the mouth as the baby sucks and closes the opening.

A child with this defect cannot speak plainly and usually an effort is made to remedy it by an operation when it is time for it to learn to talk. Great care in training the voice is necessary that the tones may be pleasant.

Tongue Tie

In this condition the membrane under the tongue is shortened, or misplaced, so that the tongue cannot be protruded beyond the teeth. The child cannot nurse and makes a clucking noise in trying to do so. The obstruction can easily be snipped by a surgeon. This should not be attempted by anyone else, as in some cases the cutting may be followed by serious bleeding. Ordinarily, it is a very trivial operation.

If it is not attended to, it will interfere with distinctness of speech as the child grows older.

Birthmarks

Very few children are born without some blemish or imperfection of the skin. Usually these are so unimportant that they are almost unnoticed. Many disappear after a time and, if not, give so little trouble that they are seldom thought of even by those who bear them.

When they appear on the face or in other conspicuous positions, they may cause great annoyance, and, if possible, should be removed early in the child's life.

Moles, or dark spots on the skin, and port wine or fire marks are the most common. The former are usually easily dealt with; the latter are far more difficult of removal, although a skillful surgeon may not find the task a hopeless one.

In any case the best advice that can be obtained should be had, as permanent disfigurement is a thing to be avoided by any means in one's power.

Extra Fingers

Occasionally a child is born with more than the normal number of fingers or toes. The extra one can be removed with little inconvenience and, as young babies generally bear slight operations well, it is best to have it done as soon as possible. There is very little loss of blood and, under favorable conditions, the wound soon heals.

Protrusion of Navel

After the cord drops off it may be observed that the navel pouts or protrudes a little. It requires a smooth surface pressed against it for a few days to keep it in place. A wooden button mold, or large button with one side rounded, answers the purpose very well. It must be folded in a piece of linen and can be held in position by a piece of elastic about three inches wide with a strip of cotton sewed to each end. These should be about three inches wide also and long enough to reach nearly but not quite around the body. Eyelet holes can be worked in each end and a cord passed through them and fasten it and adjust the pressure. It can be removed when the child is washed and, probably, will be required only for a few days.

RUPTURE

It used to be imagined that there was great danger of rupture, or hernia, unless a child was tightly bandaged. The truth is, this rather increases the danger than lessens it. One of the weak points is the groin, where the band gives little or no support. In the act of crying the intestines, pushed downward by the unyielding band, are pressed against the weak spot and it may bring about the very accident it was intended to guard against.

Rupture may occur at the umbilicus, or navel, or just above the groin, and between the navel and the point of the breastbone. It is caused by the intestine forcing its way through a weak place in the wall of the abdomen. It can be felt as a soft mass under the skin, sometimes very small. By gentle pressure it can be slipped back into the abdomen through the opening it has made.

In umbilical hernia, a belt must be made as described for use in the protrusion of the navel, a little pad of folded cotton placed over the navel and held there by it.

The belt may have to be worn for a year, being removed only when the child is washed. By keeping the intestine from protruding the opening closes and there is no farther trouble.

In inguinal hernia, the swelling makes its appearance on the side of the abdomen just above the groin. The treatment is the same. The intestine must be returned by gentle manipulation and held in place by a proper truss. This cannot be applied too early. A rubber truss can be obtained, which is not injured by being wet.

Great care is necessary to keep the parts underneath it in good condition. They must be wiped with a damp cloth, carefully dried and powdered each time the napkin is changed.

The truss itself needs careful attention. It should be washed with a weak solution of carbolic acid once a day and washed and dried every time it is taken off before replacing it. A truss often has to be worn for several years and should not be discarded until the child has been inspected by a physician.

Rupture occurs in older children, particularly boys, from lifting heavy weight, or straining themselves some other way. As soon as it shows itself a truss should be provided and worn continuously.

A rupture is a comparatively simple matter as long as the intestine can be returned to the abdomen and kept there. When it is above the navel a belt like that for umbilical hernia can be worn, the pad being placed over the point of rupture.

The danger lies in not being able to return the intestine to the abdomen. In this case the child may be put in a warm bath to relax the tension. After this, he may be placed on the back with the feet higher than the head and the mass gently pressed and manipulated in the hope of being able to slip it back through the opening.

If this cannot be effected, the doctor should be sent for as the hernia may become strangulated; that is, the folds of the intestine compressed so tightly that the circulation is cut off. Obstinate vomiting and extreme depression follow and if not relieved the child dies.

The possibility of this accident renders the proper care of rupture very important.

PROLAPSE OF THE BOWEL

If a child strains too violently in the effort to have a movement the lower part of the rectum may come out beyond the anus, presenting an appearance as a soft, red tumor, very alarming to the mother if she does not know the cause of it.

If it is slight, it can easily be returned by gently pressing it back with the finger covered with a little Vaseline. When it is more severe a flannel wrung out of hot water can be applied to relax the parts before pressure is used.

The accident sometimes happens after prolonged diarrhea, or when there is constipation. The diet should be regulated and in the latter case a laxative or an enema be given before the next movement.

PILES

Piles, or hemorrhoids, are not common in young children, although they do appear and older ones suffer from them. External piles are small swelling, or tumors, appearing around the opening of the bowel. They do not bleed but when inflamed are very painful. They should be sponged with very hot or cold water, whichever gives most relief. Rest in bed is beneficial and strict attention to regularity of the bowels, as they are often due to constipation. A flannel band worn over the abdomen is also of use.

Elizabeth Robinson Scovil *The Care of Children*

Internal piles, situated farther up the passage, sometimes bleed, particularly after a movement. When this is the case, a physician should be consulted. As much as a tablespoon of blood may be lost at one time, which has a depressing effect if it is often repeated.

If internal piles descend after a movement. The finger should be covered with Vaseline and the piles gently pressed back again. An astringent ointment may be needed.

ENLARGED GLANDS

A system of glands called the lymphatic glands extends over the whole body. They are especially numerous in the neck, the groins and under the arms. Usually they cannot be felt, but when they are enlarged they are like a chain of beads to the touch. The enlargement may take place as the result of an injury, or be due to some irritation, as in teething, catarrh, or acute disease, as scarlet fever. In children with a tendency to scrofula the glands often break down, the swelling ending in the formation of matter, or pus.

The treatment in cases where the glands are enlarged is to remove or alleviate the source of irritation, if possible, give nourishing food and, if necessary, cod-liver oil.

Saltwater sponge baths are recommended and special attention should be paid to having the child warmly clad.

The glands can be painted with tincture of iodine. Bathing with hot water may give relief if they are painful. If there is heat and throbbing, pus is forming and a doctor should be consulted. When the abscess is lanced in time, the scar is smaller than if it were left to break of itself.

ENLARGEMENT OF TONSILS

Delicate children often suffer from an enlargement of the tonsils, the almond-shaped glands on each side of the entrance to the throat.

Snoring and starting or crying out in the sleep sometimes due to this cause, as well as cough.

On looking in the mouth these bodies are seen to be swelled, projecting towards each other, as the tonsils have a tendency to decrease in size with increasing age. If they interfere with nursing, as in a young baby, or cause much discomfort, home treatment will be of little avail unless carried out under the direction of a physician.

When matter forms in the tonsils and they discharge, we have the condition known as quinsy. At this stage poultices are applied externally and every means adopted to hasten the suppuration. In aggravated cases it is necessary to remove the whole or a part of the gland.

The directions as to food, baths and clothing in enlargement of the other glands should be followed. It is especially necessary that farinaceous food, as oatmeal, bread, etc., should be limited, milk and meat being increased.

WARTS

Erasmus Wilson, one of the great authorities on diseases of the skin, says that warts are caused by some interference with the nutrition of the skin. This is more or less under the control of the nervous system, which accounts for the disappearance of warts under the influence of charms, that act upon the mind alone. Constitutional treatment, as tonics and nourishing food, may be required if the warts are numerous or persistent.

A good application is:

Salicylic Acid, one dram,
Lactic Acid, one dram,
Flexible Collodion, two drams.
Mix and apply with a camel-hair brush twice a day.

FRECKLES

Children with fair skin, particularly if the hair is red, freckle very easily. The face should be protected as much as possible by a wide-brimmed hat. Persistent washing with buttermilk of the parts affected will remove them. If this cannot be obtained, lactic acid diluted with one-half water may be substituted. It is this acid that gives the buttermilk its virtue.

TAN

Tan is rather becoming than otherwise to most children. If it is desired to remove the brown coloring it can be done by covering the surface thickly with benzoate zinc ointment at night and washing it with soap and hot water in the morning.

SUNBURN

The smarting of sunburn is relieved by bathing with vinegar followed by a copious application of cold cream.

A BLUE BABY

The condition of cyanosis, as it is technically called, which causes a baby to look blue, arises from some affection of the heart. In severe cases the child lives only a short time, a few hours or days. Otherwise, with care, its life may be prolonged for years.

Elizabeth Robinson Scovil *The Care of Children*

Careful attention to diet, warmth and fresh air are especially necessary.

The baby should be laid on the right side. When the breathing is oppressed, it just be supported in a sitting position. If there is much distress it can be placed in a warm salt-water bath and five or six drops of brandy given, the dose being repeated once or twice, until the doctor can see it.

As the child grows older the diet must consist of milk, meat, bread, vegetables and farinaceous food, all rich or indigestible articles of diet being scrupulously avoided.

Flannel must be worn next the skin and the feet protected with especial care.

Warm water must always be used for bathing, and in very cold weather the child should stay indoors.

Cold is the enemy to be dreaded above all others. At the same time ventilation of the sleeping room is most important.

A child suffering in this way should not be allowed to take violent exercise, nor over-exert himself in any way. The studies just be regulated not to overtax the brain.

The child is really an invalid, yet one who should be encouraged to make the most of his powers while being extremely careful not to exceed them.

DISEASES OF CHILDREN
CHAPTER XXI

THE EARLY STAGES

The watchful mother will be on the alert to detect the first symptoms of illness of her child. Loss of appetite, languor and fretfulness should always arouse suspicion.

An ailing child should not be allowed to sleep in the same room with those who are well and should as far as possible be separated from them until the nature of the illness is known. Some of the contagious diseases are infectious in the very early stages.

Vomiting, not caused by indigestible food, diarrhea, or rapid rise of temperature, are all reasons for keeping the child in bed and on light diet, as milk diluted with lime water, a little bread and gruel, until farther symptoms have declared themselves.

The throat should be looked at, the face, neck and body carefully examined for traces of a rash, and any complaint of pain attended to and remembered for the doctor's information.

If there is anything unusual about the discharges they should be saved in a covered vessel for the doctor's inspection and kept out of doors if possible. The mother must remember that it is often difficult for him to make a diagnosis in the obscure case, or early in the disease, and she may be able to throw much light on the subject by telling him of symptoms that seem to her unimportant.

POINTS OF NURSING
VENTILATION

The sick room must be ventilated. Pure air must be admitted from the outside and warm air supplied to keep the temperature at 60°F – 65°F in fevers, at 68°F in chronic diseases, and 70°F in diseases of the chest and respiratory tract.

Poisonous matter is constantly being thrown off by the skin and lungs, and if this poison remains in the room it is reabsorbed by the system and does almost as much harm as if it were poison administered by mouth with a teaspoon.

A safe way of admitting fresh air, when cold is to be especially guarded against, is to keep the window in an adjoining room, or the hall, open, and to air the sick room from it. The air can then be tempered by artificial hear before it enters the apartment of the invalid.

Cooling the Sick Room

In very hot weather the openings of the windows can be covered with cloths dipped into cold or iced water. The door should be left open and if necessary, a fan used to set the air in the room in motion. In India, bamboo or grass screens, kept wet by being sprayed or dashed with water, are used for this purpose. The temperature of the room can be perceptibly lowered by this means. The heated air is cooked by passing through the damp medium.

Furniture

Unnecessary article of furniture should be removed, and all remain wiped every day with a damp cloth.

The Carpet

In serious illness the carpet should be taken up. Where this is impossible a square of linen should be spread under the bed and carefully wiped off every morning with a cloth squeezed out of carbolic solution, 1 – 40. The carpet itself should be brushed with a carpet sweeper, or, if this is too noisy, a broom with a bag drawn over it, moistened with disinfectant.

The Screen

A screen should be provided to guard the eyes from the light, and sunlight admitted to the room, unless in disease of the brain, smallpox, or when the eyes are weak, as in measles.

The Bed

The bed should be protected with a square of India-rubber cloth under the sheet. If it is folded in a sheet placed crossways of the bed, it can be removed when soiled without disturbing the under sheet.

When the temperature is high cover lightly with one thin blanket. If a light of white spread is not at hand use a sheet instead.

Changing Clothing

In changing the night dress draw it up in the back until the folds lie under the neck, lay the arms above the head on the pillow, slip the night dress over the head from behind, then draw it off the arms.

In putting on the clean one fit the sleeves of the under shirt into those of the night dress and they will go on as one garment. Put the arms on first, then raising them as before slip the night dress over the head and draw it down smoothly under the back. Clean clothing should always be aired and warmed. When moving is difficult, have the night dress open all the way down an put it on like an apron.

Nutritive Enemata

When food cannot be given by mouth or retained in the stomach, it is necessary to administer it by enema. The points to be remembered are that the bowel must first be washed out by an enema of warm water. The nutritive enema must be about the temperature of the body, not hotter than 99°F, small in quantity, not exceeding two or three ounces, four or six tablespoonfuls, or one tablespoonful for a young baby, and given slowly, or it will not be retained.

The best instrument to use a rectal tube, a rubber tube about fifteen inches long, pointed at one end and with a funnel attached at the other.

Vaseline the pointed end, insert it gently into the rectum as far as possible, raise the funnel and pour the fluid slowly into it. Press the tube gently with the fingers from the rectum towards the funnel to press the air out, if the fluid does not flow in readily.

A bulb syringe may be used but must be squeezed very slowly and carefully.

Milk, white of egg, beef juice and sometimes brandy or whiskey, are used.

The milk and beef juice should be peptonized, or pre-digested. In the case of beef juice this can be done by the following recipe:

Peptonized Beef Juice

Mince half a pound of lean raw beef, add ten grains of pepsin and two drops of hydrochloric acid and cover with cold water. Place the jar in water of 90°F and let it remain at this temperature for two hours.

Nutritive enemata must not be given more often than once in four hours. The bowel should be cleansed with an enema of plain warm water every twenty-four hours.

Forced Feeding, or Gavage

When a child vomits persistently, or refuses to take food in serious illness, it is sometimes administered by passing a tube down the throat and pouring the food in. It is not nearly as distressing a method as forcing a child to take food from a spoon when it struggles against doing so and resists violently, and is much more effectual, as the nourishment goes into the stomach without the exhaustions that follow resistance.

The apparatus is a soft rubber catheter with a double eye, a short glass tube to connect the catheter with eighteen inches of rubber tubing and a small funnel.

The child is laid on the back, the tongue held down with a finger, and the point of the catheter passed down the throat about ten inches, keeping it well to the back of the mouth.

The funnel is held high up to allow gas to escape from the stomach, and then the food poured in, three or four ounces being given, according to the age of the child. Peptonized milk is generally used. If the mouth is held open for a few minutes after the catheter is withdrawn the child is less likely to vomit.

The stomach should be washed out with plain boiled water once a day.

After using, the tubes must be thoroughly washed in a solution of baking soda in water, it being poured through them again and again, and well-rinsed in clear, warm water. About once in three days the apparatus must be boiled.

A glass funnel is the best to use, although a tin or hard rubber one will answer the purpose if it is kept exquisitely clean. Unless properly attended to, the tubes may become a distinct source of danger.

Poultices

Flaxseed mean is the best material for a poultice. A cupful is sufficient for a medium-sized one. Have the water boiling in a saucepan; stir in the meal gradually; when it is boiled a minute take it from the fire and beat it thoroughly to make it light. If too thin boil it down a little. It should spread easily but not run. Have ready a piece of cotton the size of the poultice desired, spread the flaxseed on it, leaving a border an inch wide on every side; lay over it an old handkerchief, fold the edges of both upon the poultice like a hem, and it is ready.

Be careful not to apply it too hot, as the skin of a child is tender, and bandage it in place with a towel or piece of cotton. If it is covered with a sheet of wadding or double fold of flannel it will keep hot longer.

Fomentations

It is easy to wring flannels out of boiling water without burning the fingers, if one knows how.

Place a dry towel over a basin, lay the folded flannel on it, pour over it the boiling water. Taking the towel by the dry ends fold it over the flannel and, by twisting the ends in opposite directions, it can be wrung dry without wetting the hands.

Shake out the flannel before applying it, as a little air between the folds prevents the heat from escaping so rapidly. Cover with a piece of India-rubber cloth or a thick newspaper.

Pads

When for any reason the discharges are involuntary, pads will be found a great comfort, as they render the little sufferer more comfortable and save much washing.

Take several thicknesses of newspaper, place on this a layer of oakum, cotton waste, or any soft absorbent substance, and cover the whole with cheese cloth or old cotton. When it is soiled it can be rolled up and burned. A square of rubber cloth, or table oil cloth, can be used as a foundation, being carefully sponged with disinfectant each time the pad is changed.

Soiled napkins, pads, or vessels containing discharges should not be allowed to remain in any room where there are children, sick or well, for longer than it takes to remove them. Every mother should make this an invariable rule.

Preventing Infection

Isolation of the patient and nurse and thorough disinfection of everything that leaves the sick room will prevent the spread of the infection.

A room in the top story should be chosen if possible and all communication with the rest of the house forbidden. Whatever is to be brought to the sick room should be left outside the door and everything to be taken away put in the same place. When the nurse leaves the room she should rub her hair thoroughly with a clean towel, kept outside the room, change her wrapper for a fresh one, wash her face and hands, and put on another pair of shoes.

Disinfectants

Many disinfectants are recommended and, no doubt, are good. Any disease can be prevented from spreading by the use of carbolic acid for general purposes, sulphate of zinc and common salt for the clothing, and lime, or copperas, for the water closet.

It is the cheapest to buy the pure carbolic acid in crystals. Stand the bottle in hot water and the crystals become liquid; mix one part to twenty of water for putting in the vessels in which the discharges are received and dilute this solution one-half for washing the hands, wiping the furniture, etc.

The lotion recommended for the chapped hands will keep the hands smooth and soft while using the disinfectant.

For the clothing, add a quarter of a pound of sulphate of zinc and half as much salt to a gallon of hot water. Soak the clothes in this and have them boiled in the laundry in water to which washing soda has been added. If this is not done, the clothes will have a disagreeable, greasy feeling after they are dried.

Elizabeth Robinson Scovil *The Care of Children*

A pail of water with as much copperas in it as it will dissolve should be poured down the closet each time it is used. If there is not a water closet a thick layer of lime should be put in the closet with a shovel instead.

FUMIGATION

At the close of the illness at least two pounds of Sulphur should be burned in the room, the doors and windows being tightly closed. Furniture should be washed in carbolic acid, stuffed furniture and mattresses being first fumigated, then the covers burned, and the upholstery removed.

Walls and ceilings must be scrubbed, repapered, painted or lime-washed, as they may require. Every article that cannot be cleansed must be burned. The danger is too great to justify running any avoidable risk.

Sulphur candles can be obtained which are more convenient than the powdered Sulphur. When this is used a crumpled newspaper should be put in an old coalscuttle, or iron pan, and the Sulphur sprinkled on it. The iron receptacle can be stood in a tub containing water to prevent any danger of fire. The newspaper is lighted, and the room closed as quickly as possible.

Moisture is very necessary to make the gas dis-engaged from the burning Sulphur effective. The walls and floor should be sprinkled with water and all surfaces that can be reached wetted.

SCARLET FEVER
SYMPTOMS

Sore throat; sometimes a rash may be seen on the tonsils and back of the throat before it appears on the skin. Vomiting is common.

RASH

Bright scarlet, in small points, does not feel raised to the touch, appears first on the upper part of the chest and about the lower part of the neck, extending to the arms.

The tongue presents a peculiar appearance known as the "strawberry tongue". It is coated with a whitish fur through which pink points project.

PROGRESS

There is usually high fever and thirst; water may be given and weak lemonade. Towards the end of the first week the rash begins to fade, and desquamation commences. The skin peels off, sometimes in small particles, sometimes in large flakes. This process lasts for a week or ten days, and often much longer on the hands and feet. The fever should decline when peeling begins.

POINTS TO BE OBSERVED

If the urine decreases in quantity disease of the kidneys may be feared. Earache, or discharge from the ear, should be reported to the doctor, as the inflammation may have extended from the throat to the ear through the eustachian tube, or passage connecting them. Puffiness about the eyes must be watched for.

NURSING

Free ventilation is extremely important, yet cold, or a sudden chill, may cause dangerous complications. The room must not be colder than 65°F. A sponge bath is given every day under a blanket; sometimes more often if the temperature is high.

During desquamation the body is anointed with carbolized Vaseline or benzoinated lard, followed by a sponge bath of warm water with a little washing soda dissolved in it, to allay the irritation and disinfect the particles of skin by means of which the contagion is conveyed to others.

All clothing must be warmed before being put on. Liquid food is ordered and should be given every two hours.

If pulse and temperature should fall suddenly, teaspoonful doses of brandy may be given every ten minutes for four or five doses until the doctor can be obtained, and heat is applied.

PERIOD OF INFECTION

The patient may be disinfected in six weeks from the beginning of the disease, if peeling has ceased.

The entire person must be bathed and the hair thoroughly washed with a saturated solution of boracic acid, followed by a bath of warm water and soap.

Clean clothing that has not been in the sick room must be put on.

Children between two and seven years of age are peculiarly liable to the disease. A child who has been exposed may develop it at any time from a few hours to twenty-one days.

It is very infectious in certain cases. Others may come in close contact with it, yet escape unharmed.

It is said not to be infectious until the throat symptoms have appeared.

A very malignant case may develop from exposure to very light one.

The virulence of the disease depends not so much on the germ which

Elizabeth Robinson Scovil *The Care of Children*

communicates it as on the soil into which the germ falls. Conditions may exist in one child which will cause a severe attack from the same poison that in another child would produce only mild symptoms of the malady.

Too much care cannot be exercised in isolation and disinfection. The mattress used should always be burned.

There should be the same watchfulness in a light case as in a severe one in the avoidance of cold. Dangerous complications may follow any imprudence, even when the child does not seem very ill.

Scarlatina is the Latin name of the disease and not a milder form.

Scarlet Rash is the same dread enemy and equally to be feared.

MEASLES
SYMPTOMS

A cold in the head with discharge from the nose and inflamed eyes. After three days of languor and feverishness the rash appears on the fourth day in dots, feeling rough under the skin. It is first seen on the forehead, about the hair and on the cheek bones. Sometimes the blotches are half-moon-shaped and are of a dark red color.

There may be nausea, vomiting and a cough.

PROGRESS

The disease should reach its height about the sixth day, remain stationary for two days and then the patient should begin to improve. At its height the rash covers the whole body and there may be high fever.

POINTS TO BE OBSERVED

The points of danger are the eyes and chest. If the watery discharge from the eyes is succeeded by matter or pus, the doctor should be informed.

Should the cough increase, the breathing become difficult, or pain in the chest be complained of; warm camphorated oil must be rubbed on the chest covered with flannel until the physician comes.

There is a fine, mealy desquamation, but not as marked as the peeling in scarlet fever.

NURSING

The room must be darkened on account of the eyes. The child should not be permitted to use them even during convalescence.

While ventilation is very important, the room must be kept warm on account of the danger to the chest. About 68°F is a good temperature. Isolation and thorough disinfection are necessary.

PERIOD OF INFECTION

Measles is infectious in the very early stages, as soon as the symptoms of cold appear, until the rash is gone, and the cough has ceased; usually about three weeks from its commencement.

If a child exposed to it does not develop the disease in between seven and twenty-one days after exposure it has probably escaped. It is said that babies under six months rarely take measles or scarlet fever.

GERMAN MEASLES

The mother may confound this rash with either measles or scarlet fever, and sometimes the characteristic scarlet fever tongue is present.

It usually comes on very suddenly, the child awaking in the morning covered with rash, having been apparently quite well the night before. There may be a little sore throat, but the fever is very slight, if there is any. The glands at the back of the neck are tender, and this point helps to decide in distinguishing the disease.

Little treatment is needed. The child should be kept indoors and in bed if the throat is sore. A gentle laxative may be needed. The disappearance of the rash means an end of the trouble.

CHICKEN POX
SYMPTOMS

The eruption of chicken pox usually appears on the upper part of the back or chest first, though sometimes on the face. It begins as small red spots, which change to little vesicles, containing a watery fluid. On the second or third day they commence to dry up, a scab forming over them. If they are scratched they may leave white scars behind which never disappear.

The child is feverish for a few days and should be kept in bed if this condition is marked. A tonic may be required if there is languor and want of appetite after the vesicles are healed.

Elizabeth Robinson Scovil *The Care of Children*

The disease can be communicated until the scabs have all dropped off. Three weeks is the longest period they persist. Eighteen days after exposure the child may be considered safe if it has not developed.

Disinfection is not necessary, as it is such a mild disorder.

VACCINATION

The English law required that babies shall be vaccinated before they are three months old, unless a medical certificate can be obtained to certify that they are suffering from some malady or weakness, that renders the operation undesirable or improper.

In many States of the Union children cannot be admitted to the public schools until they have been vaccinated.

If as slight an operation as this can protect a child from the possibility of suffering disfigurement or death from smallpox, it seems wrong not to have it performed.

Many parents shrink from having it done because they fear that other diseases may be communicated by the inoculation.

Within the last twenty years vaccinating young cattle to produce the vaccine lymph has been followed as a business, and this virus can be obtained in good condition, rendering the use of that from human beings unnecessary.

The outside of the thigh is a better place for vaccination than the arm. The doctor scratches the surface or cuts a number of fine lines on it with a lancet, and rubs in the vaccine. It is an almost painless operation.

In about three days it begins to take, and in about eight or nine is at its height. There is a pustule surrounded with a rim of inflamed surface that often itches.

There may be a little fever and some constitutional disturbance. This gradually subsides and in three weeks nothing remains but the scar to tell the tale.

An unvaccinated child exposed to smallpox should be vaccinated immediately, as the vaccine virus acts more quickly than the small-pox poison and helps to neutralize it.

It is considered best to have it done before the baby is four months old, that the disturbance may be over before the teething begins.

DIPHTHERIA

This is one of the most alarming diseases of childhood. It is now said that it can only be determined whether a disease is true diphtheria or not by a microscopical examination of the exudation to discover the germ that causes it. This being the case it is wise to treat all suspicious cases as if they were indeed the dreaded foe, that no carelessness may give cause for future reproach.

Dampness and want of cleanliness in cellars and sleeping rooms forms a favorable soil for the growth of poison causing diphtheria. Bad ventilation predisposes to it; sewer gas, infected with the germ, carries it with deadly certainty.

Symptoms

These may at first be very slight, headache, languor and feverishness, with nothing to distinguish them from those of an ordinary cold.

Whenever a child complains of illness the throat should be examined and, if it is sore, a physician sent for.

The patches of membrane in diphtheria appear on the tonsils, and extend to the surrounding parts. They can usually be seen on the folds of membrane on each side of the throat forming the arch at the back of the mouth. There is difficulty in swallowing, which sometimes first calls attention to the throat.

When there is tonsilitis, or inflammation of the tonsils, they are covered with yellowish white spots, but these come off easily, if touched with a camel's-hair brush dipped in compound tincture of benzoin. The diphtheritic membrane adheres closely and is removed with difficulty.

Progress

The case may be very mild or very severe. There is no more treacherous disease than this. Its duration is uncertain and constant watchfulness is needed.

Points to be Observed

If the voice becomes husky, or the breathing labored, the physician should be informed. The heart is affected, and, if the pulse becomes feeble and the feet cold, heat should be applied to the extremities and a teaspoonful of brandy given.

It is always well in serious illness to ask the doctor what emergencies are likely to arise and the measures that may be taken to meet them, as time is often lost before he can be found.

The child should be kept lying down and not permitted to sit up for any purpose. Small bed pans and urinals can be purchased that render sitting-up unnecessary.

Squares of soft cotton, or old linen, should be used to receive the discharge from the nose and mouth. These must be sprinkled with disinfectant, rolled in newspaper and burned.

Elizabeth Robinson Scovil *The Care of Children*

Bits of ice may be given. The food must be nourishing and concentrated on account of the difficulty in swallowing. Albuminized milk, beef juice, strong mutton broth, yolk of eggs with brandy, when stimulant is given, and malted milk. If the digestion is impaired the milk can be sterilized, or peptonized. The applications ordered for the throat have to be applied, although sometimes it is a very distressing task. Spray thrown with an atomizer is more effectual and less likely to injure the parts than applications made with a brush.

PERIOD OF INFECTION

As the disease is very infectious, the child must be isolated and thorough disinfection and fumigation follow the termination of the case.

If other children in the family are exposed to the same influences as the patient was they may contract the disease even though they do not get it from him. If they are removed from the house and it does not develop within twelve days, they probably have escaped.

The invalid should be kept in quarantine for six weeks from the beginning of the attack and only released if there is no sore throat nor other symptom of the disease.

CROUP

There are two varieties of croup, membranous and spasmodic. The first, or true croup, is considered by many authorities as identical with diphtheria. The symptoms are the same, with the addition of sharp, hoarse cough.

It is the second, or false croup, that causes so much alarm to mothers, and this is almost never fatal.

SYMPTOMS

The child may have a hoarse cough during the day with a feeling of tightness across the chest towards night. There may be no cough, the head and hands feeling a little hot. With or without previous symptoms, the child wakens in the night with a croupy cough and often breathing with great difficulty.

Hot fomentations, flannels wrung out of boiling water, should be applied to the throat and, if fleece nary, a warm bath given. Anything that will relax the parts will do good.

If the distress continues, vomiting will give relief. Teaspoonful doses of wine of ipecac may be given, of the same quantity of powdered alum stirred into syrup, molasses or jam. These should be followed by draughts of tepid water.

If the hoarseness comes on in the afternoon ten drops of win of ipecac, repeated every half hour until the child feels a little nauseated, may prevent an attack.

Children subject to croup should be kept indoors on damp days, wear flannel undergarments, have the feet well protected and, as far as possible, be prevented from screaming to strain the vocal chords. The throat should be bathed with cold water every morning and thoroughly rubbed afterwards with the hand.

WHOOPING COUGH
Symptoms

The early symptoms of whooping cough are like those of a bad cold and is difficult to speak positively as to its existence until the characteristic whoop is heard, although in young babies this is sometimes absent.

The paroxysms are often very severe. There is a succession of short coughs with not opportunity to breathe between them, until the child seems on the point of suffocating, there is a long-drawn inspiration with the whistling sound that gives the disease its name, and the lungs fill again. If the sufferer is old enough, he spits out a thick, tenacious mucus.

The fit of coughing may cause vomiting, or bleeding from the nose. In the latter case the blood is sometimes swallowed and appears later as a black, tarry mass in the motions, or, being retained in the stomach, returns with the vomitus after the next attack.

It need not cause alarm. There is very seldom sufficient bleeding from the lungs to warrant anxiety, and blood from that quarter is always bright red and mixed with little bubbles of air.

Progress

After two weeks the paroxysms should be less frequent. The cough may last for two months or longer.

Points to be Observed

If there is vomiting, food should be given every three hours in smaller quantities than usual, choosing the time immediately after a fit of coughing that it may be retained as long as possible. Tonics and cod-liver oil may be needed.

At night the bed should be covered with a mosquito netting, as a draught is very apt to bring on the cough.

Elizabeth Robinson Scovil *The Care of Children*

The chest should be carefully protected with an extra fold of flannel and rubbed back and front twice a day with warm oil.

Steaming the throat with thirty drops of pure carbolic acid in two and one-half pints of boiling water is said to be an excellent remedy. The water is put in a hot pitcher and the child's head held over it; both being covered with a towel to confine the steam. It may be repeated three to four times a day.

The patient may go out on warm, dry days, taking care that he is not brough in contact with other children. Cold increases the violence of the cough.

PERIOD OF INFECTION

Whooping cough is an extremely infectious disease and easily communicated from one child to another. Those suffering from it should be isolated and not allowed to travel in cars, play in parks, or mix with others who have not had the disease. The danger is not over until the cough has entirely ceased.

It is said that it can be conveyed by means of clothing, or playthings, worn or used by the little patient, and all such should be carefully disinfected.

If a child who has been exposed to it does not exhibit the symptoms within three weeks he has probably escaped.

MUMPS

This painful disease is an inflammation of the parotid glands immediately below the ear at the angle of the jaw. Sometimes only one side is affected and sometimes both. The disease is apt to occur again if only one side is involved.

SYMPTOMS

A swelling appears below the ear accompanied by slight fever, general depression and loss of appetite. Opening the mouth is difficult and an acid, as vinegar, causes an intense pain to shoot through the affected part.

PROGRESS

Occasionally, when one side is nearly well, the other swells, thus lengthening the attack.

The swelling may attack other glands and this metastasis, as it is called, may be caused by cold.

It is well to keep the child in bed, or if not sufficiently uncomfortable for this, at least to confine him to one warm, well-ventilated room.

Chewing is so painful that the diet must consist of milk, eggs, and soup.

A laxative may be given if there is constipation. When there are no complications, the attack only lasts a week or ten days.

PERIOD OF INFECTION

A child who has been exposed to the disease may develop it at any time between six days and two weeks. Usually, the incubation is about a week. After three weeks he may be considered absolutely safe.

TYPHOID FEVER

Typhoid fever is propagated by a germ which may be conveyed in water, or milk, or taken into the system by other means. It is said by many authorities that it must be swallowed, not merely breathed in. The disease is most common in autumn, following a hot, dry summer.

The small intestine is ulcerated. One of the points of danger lies in these ulcers penetrating the intestine and causing fatal inflammation. To avoid this the diet must be strictly regulated and the child kept as quiet as possible.

SYMPTOMS

The little invalid seems indisposed to play, the legs ache and headache, particularly in the forehead, is complained of. The sleep is restless and there is usually constipation, although diarrhea may be present. The thermometer shows a rise of temperature in the evening, falling again in the morning.

There is little appetite and much thirst.

PROGRESS

Often during the second week a crop of rose-colored spots appear on the abdomen, the lower part of the chest and between the shoulder-blades.

The mother should watch for these and report their appearance to the doctor.

There should be improvement at the end of the third week and convalescence begin by the close of the fourth.

POINTS TO BE OBSERVED

The lips are apt to be dry and cracked and the teeth covered with an accumulation called sordes. They should be frequently cleansed with a little lemon juice and glycerin and the lips kept moist with glycerin or Vaseline.

Elizabeth Robinson Scovil *The Care of Children*

BED SORES

There is a special pre-disposition to bed sores wherever pressure comes on the body, as the lower part of the back, the shoulders, heels and elbows.

These parts should be bathed morning and evening with alcohol and well rubbed and powdered with French chalk. The rubbing is all-important to promote circulation. A bed sore will not form when this is faithfully done.

The parts should be examined several times during the twenty-four hours and wherever the slightest trace of redness is perceived it should be chafed and rubbed until it has disappeared.

If a bed sore forms, it must be relieved from pressure by means of a rubber ring, washed with carbolized water 1-100 and dressed with balsam of Peru, or some healing salve.

FOOD

The food must be liquid, milk and limewater, albuminized milk, broths if the doctor permits, kumis, etc.

If the digestion is impaired the milk can be peptonized.

Plenty of water is given to drink and must be offered if not asked for. Weak lemonade, barley water, or a little fruit syrup in the water may be more readily taken. The food must be given regularly every two hours. When there is great distaste for it, only a small quantity need be administered. Solid food must not be ventured on until the temperature has been normal for a week, nor then without the doctor's express permission. Neglect of this precaution may cause death.

INFECTION

While typhoid fever is not infectious in the ordinary sense of the word, it can be communicated through the movements. All discharges, including the water, should be received in a vessel containing carbolic acid 1-20, covered with it before being emptied and the water closet deluged with copperas solution. If the excretions are disinfected thoroughly, the disease cannot spread. In the country it is best to mix them with sawdust and burn them.

When they are thrown away without proper disinfection, they may filter into pure water contaminating it so that those who drink it may take the disease.

In one instance an epidemic is said to have originated from the use of milk which had been put into cans washed in water impregnated with the poisonous germs.

It is important that those who are nursing a case of typhoid fever should disinfect the hands before eating.

PNEUMONIA

Pneumonia, or inflammation of the lungs, is said to be one of the most common of the more severe diseases of childhood and most often occurs between four and seven years of age. Good authorities assert that it may be caused by foul air, as the escape of sewer gas into a house, as well as by cold.

SYMPTOMS

It comes on suddenly with vomiting followed by very high fever and runs its course in five or six days, the child recovering rapidly, or the illness terminating fatally.

The breathing is rapid, the nostrils dilating with each respiration and the pulse very quick. There is cough and a deep flush on one or both cheeks. The child refuses food but may take a little milk, milk and Vichy, or milk with lime water. Not much nourishment is needed during the short time the fever lasts. It cannot be digested, and the child will not sink from exhaustion for want of it. The physician will order stimulant if it is required.

POINTS TO BE OBSERVED

If there is reason to suspect that the plumbing is defective, the child should be removed from the house to a purer atmosphere.

Ventilation is always important; the temperature being kept about 68°F. It is important that it should not vary.

When the fever is high, careful sponging with tepid water under a blanket is desirable. Frequent bathing of hands and face is soothing.

A flannel jacket should be worn over the night dress as the child has to be supported with pillows in a half-sitting position to breathe comfortably.

The chest is rubbed with warm oil and protected with flannel or cotton batting.

BRONCHITIS

A cold on the chest is really a light attack of bronchitis. The bronchial tubes, which conduct air from the windpipe to the lungs are inflamed, the delicate lining membrane being very susceptible in some persons. Living in heated rooms and breathing too warm dry air predisposes to it. Children and old persons are especially liable to it, and it is more apt to be fatal in them than in others. Exposure to a cold wind with the chest insufficiently protected may bring it on in a child. When it attacks the smaller branches of the tubes it is called capillary bronchitis, and this is an especially dangerous form.

Elizabeth Robinson Scovil *The Care of Children*

SYMPTOMS

Those of cold on the chest, with feverishness, hoarseness, more or less pain in the upper part of the chest and a slight cough. A child is usually especially languid and depressed. Young children almost always swallow the sputa; if it can be seen, it is at first watery, then thick and sticky.

TREATMENT

The room must be kept at an even temperature of about 68°F. Moisture can be introduced into the air by keeping a kettle boiling if there is a fire, or by a large sponge or cloth wrung out of water and allowed to dry over the register, or radiator, being re-wet as often as necessary.

The throat may be steamed over a pitcher of boiling water with one teaspoonful of spirits of turpentine in it, or thirty drops of tincture of benzoin.

A mustard paste can be applied over the chest, or flaxseed poultices, changed every hour. After these applications are removed it may be rubbed with warm oil and covered with flannel.

Hot lemonade, flaxseed tea, or any warm soothing drink is beneficial. The food should be especially nourishing.

A young child who is seriously ill with bronchitis should not be allowed to sleep too long at one time for fear of the secretions accumulating in the tubes, or collecting at the back of the mouth, in such quantity that they cannot be disposed of.

The disease may pass into the chronic stage. The child always has a slight cough in cold weather, and it may persist into the summer. It does not thrive and gain flesh as it should do. Sometimes removal to a milder climate will effect a cure. There is always danger of an acute attack developing. Children in this condition should have special care as to clothing and food and be kept indoors in cold or damp weather.

ASTHMA

Asthma is a spasmodic contraction of the bronchial tubes, causing at times great difficulty in breathing. There is sometimes an inherited tendency to the affection, one of the parents having been similarly afflicted. Sometimes it is caused by dust, or the odor from certain plants, or animals. It may follow bronchitis, whooping cough, or measles, or be caused by anger, fright, indigestion, or constipation, and seems to be brought on by any cause that inflames the membrane lining the bronchial tubes.

SYMPTOMS

The child is often wakened from sleep by the difficulty of breathing. The symptoms are much the same as those of false croup. The distinction is said to be, that in croup there is a struggle to draw the breath in, and in asthma to exhale, or breathe out. The paroxysm may last from half an hour to a much longer time.

TREATMENT

This, during the paroxysm, is much the same as in croup. Inhalations of the steam from very hot water; hot fomentations to the throat and ten to fifteen drop doses of wine of ipecac, repeated four, or five times, until the child is a little nauseated. The object is to relax the parts and so relieve the spasm, and the condition of nausea is a very relaxing one.

Children frequently outgrow the tendency. A change of climate is desirable. Gymnastic exercises that tend to develop and strengthen the chest are valuable. Warm clothing should be worn, the feet protected, and exposure avoided.

The diet must be attended to, and the last meal of the day be of light, easily digested food. Toast or crackers should be substituted for bread, potatoes prohibited, and the cereals used in moderation, as starchy food has an unfavorable effect. Meat, fish, and eggs may be used with care, not being given later in the day than the midday meal. Milk and good soup may be partaken of freely.

RHEUMATISM

Children may inherit this disease from rheumatic parents, or contact it from exposure to a cold draught, or from being chilled while perspiring after play.

SYMPTOMS

There is a little tenderness or swelling of the joints of the wrists, knees, or ankles; sometimes the back of the knee is painful, or there is stiff neck. The temperature is apt to rise at night and there may be headache. As the heart is often involved, a physician should be consulted when rheumatism is suspected.

POINTS TO BE OBSERVED

The child must wear **a** flannel night-dress and sleep between blankets.

If the joints are painful, they can be wrapped in flannel, or cotton batting, kept in place with a light bandage. They must be propped in an easy position with pillows.

Elizabeth Robinson Scovil *The Care of Children*

Food

While the fever is high the diet is liquid; as it falls, farinaceous food, eggs and broths are given, and finally fish and meat.

Precautions

A child with rheumatic tendency should be protected from cold by warm clothing, but not kept in **a** hot room. A tepid salt-water sponge bath, followed by vigorous friction, should be given every morning. If the child is accidentally over-heated, an extra wrap should be put on until he can be undressed, sponged and rubbed.

The diet should be nourishing, avoiding too much meat. The bowels should not be allowed to become constipated, and plenty of sleep should be insisted upon.

CHOREA

This disease is commonly called St. Vitus' Dance, and girls are more often afflicted with it than boys. It is said that competition at school has been found to be one of the exciting causes.

It may also occur from fright, or follow rheumatism, or scarlet fever.

Symptoms

There is an irregular, twitching movement of the face, tongue, hands and fingers; sometimes the muscles of the legs and body are involved.

Only one side of the body may be affected, The movements cease when the child is asleep.

Children whose nerves and brain are kept on the stretch, stimulated by over-study or excitement of any kind, are apt to develop chorea.

The outlook is good if the child has proper treatment, and of this, rest is the most important.

Treatment

Study should be stopped, early hours insisted upon, and rest in bed for several hours every day enforced if the case is a severe one.

An active exercise should be forbidden, and only gradually resumed as there is a decided improvement.

While in bed, the child may be amused with simple games and allowed to read amusing, unexciting stories. Sponging with tepid water every day is valuable, if after the bath the child is wrapped in **a** blanket and persuaded to sleep.

The food should be light and nourishing—milk, eggs and gruels, with a moderate quantity of digestible solid food.

If there is sleeplessness after the hot milk and heat to the feet have been tried in vain, the doctor should be asked to prescribe.

Children who suffer from St. Vitus' Dance should never be subjected to the strain of a school examination, nor any mental excitement that can be avoided.

RICKETS

Rickets is a disease of childhood, often beginning in early infancy. It affects the general nutrition, and especially the proper development of the bones, causing deformity. It proceeds from insufficient or improper food, which cannot be digested to nourish the body. Bad ventilation, or drainage, want of sunshine and damp houses, predispose to it.

Too little milk and over-feeding with starchy food, which a baby cannot digest thoroughly, is said to be a frequent cause of rickets.

Fat alone is not an evidence of health. The muscles must be firm and the color good, the eyes bright, and the whole condition strong and vigorous to indicate that the child is well.

If the baby is nursed too long the milk ceases to satisfy the demands of the system and rickets may ensue.

Abundance of milk should be given after weaning, eggs occasionally, bread and oatmeal on account of the gluten they contain.

Symptoms

The first which the mother will observe is profuse perspiration about the head and neck as the child lies asleep. He throws off the bedclothes and seems unusually warm. Unless handled very gently he cries when he is moved or danced.

The motions are more frequent than usual, large, soft and offensive, with specks and curds of undigested food.

The fontanelle, or soft space on top of the head, which should be much smaller at the end of the first year and entirely closed before two years have passed, remains open.

If the child can walk, the legs are bowed or twisted, the wrists are enlarged, the abdomen and chest are unduly prominent, and the spine is weak and more or less curved. The teeth are late in coming.

Elizabeth Robinson Scovil *The Care of Children*

TREATMENT

The food is the first consideration. Babies under a year old should have cream in addition to the milk, raw eggs, and beef, or mutton broth. Older children must, besides these, be given meat, butter, and fresh fish, with bread, oatmeal, hominy, etc.

Cod liver oil is often prescribed as an effectual means of administering fat.

The hygienic surroundings must be attended to. Sunlight, fresh air and good ventilation, particularly of the sleeping room, being very important.

Saltwater baths have a tonic effect. Warm clothing and protection to the feet are essential.

When the child is old enough to walk he must not be permitted to do so, as permanent deformity of the legs may be caused by resting the weight on them.

Splints are sometimes worn to prevent this and keep the legs straight. The treatment recommended in bowlegs is advantageous. Sometimes a surgical operation is necessary to straighten the legs if the deformity is great.

Rickets is not necessarily fatal unless some complications ensue.

There is usually improvement as soon as the unhealthy conditions which caused it are changed.

After the errors in diet are corrected and the ventilation improved, attention should be given to the clothing. A flannel band should be worn, beside warm underclothing. This must be changed- often on account of the excessive perspiration.

The bed must be changed and aired every day and scrupulous cleanliness carried out in every particular.

The child should be kept in the open air as much as possible. If it is wheeled in a carriage a rubber hot-water bag should be placed at the feet, if the weather is at all cool.

Rubbing the body, particularly along the spine, is beneficial, and cod-liver oil applied in this way is a very useful although a disagreeable remedy.

There is hope that, as the child's condition and general nutrition improve, the deformities may lessen, if not entirely disappear.

TUBERCULOSIS

The children of consumptive parents do not necessarily inherit phthisis, or tuberculosis of the lungs. This disease is now said to be caused by a germ, or bacillus, which passes from the lungs of the infected person in the expectoration and so may communicate the malady to others.

This germ can only be carried through the air when it is dry. The sputa of persons suffering from consumption should be received into a cup containing carbolic acid 1-40, and so thoroughly disinfected before being emptied.

Squares of cotton should be carried for use in the street and burned as soon as possible after returning home. It is wrong for these persons to expectorate where the air can dry up the moisture and set the germs free to do their deadly work.

If they are breathed into the lungs of healthy persons they may do no harm, but if they come in contact with tissues predisposed to the disease, or affording a favorable soil for their growth, the mischief is done.

The utmost care should be taken to keep the belongings of consumptive persons separate from those of others. Nothing that they use should be used by anyone else without thorough cleansing.

They should not sleep with healthy persons. Kissing, or any close contact, should be discouraged.

After the death of a person from phthisis the room and its contents must be disinfected as in any other contagious disease. Upholstered furniture, as couches or easy chairs, should be fumigated with special care and re-covered.

Children with an hereditary tendency to consumption may be so built up and fortified against it by proper food and hygienic treatment, or by not being exposed to direct infection, that they may escape it altogether.

Diet is a very important factor in their case, as has been mentioned elsewhere.

Good ventilation is indispensable. Outdoor exercise in fine weather must be taken regularly.

The clothing must be warm, flannel worn and the feet protected.

Whatever tends to depress vitality, as indigestion, over-study, late hours, excess of any kind, must be avoided as far as possible.

Cod-liver oil is valuable as a good way of having fat taken. Having been elaborated in the liver of the fish it is more easily assimilated than many other forms of fat. Salt-water baths are advisable for their tonic effect.

The child's attention should not be directed towards himself nor should he be allowed to think that be is peculiarly liable to the disease.

Gymnastic exercises to strengthen and expand the chest should be practiced daily.

Tuberculosis may manifest itself in other parts than the lungs.

Sometimes the lymphatic glands in the neck are attacked and abscesses form, or *a* joint becomes the seat of a strumous, or white, swelling. The brain may be affected, causing meningitis. If the intestines are attacked ulcers form and diarrhea results, with great pain from colic.

Elizabeth Robinson Scovil *The Care of Children*

ARTICLES USEFUL IN A SICK ROOM

Urinal,
Bed pan,
Bulb syringe,
Glass syringe,
Graduated medicine glass,
Porcelain feeder,
Bent glass feeding tube,
Medicine dropper,
Rubber hot-water bag,
Rubber ice bag,
Rubber ring or cushion,
Two squares of rubber cloth,
Rubber cloth pillow case,
Granite ware basin,
Calcutta cooler for ice,
Shade for light,
Saucepan,
Alcohol lamp, or stand to fit on gas.

EMERGENCIES
CHAPTER XXII

CUTS

Cuts are amongst the most frequent accidents of childhood. A slight cut should be washed with cold water, covered with a small pad of cotton, bound up and left alone. It will usually heal without further trouble, and the dressing should not be disturbed while it is comfortable. Undoing it pulls the edges apart and interferes with the healing process.

If matter forms, or there is a disagreeable odor, the bandage must be taken off, the wound bathed with carbolized water 1-80 and a little carbolized Vaseline, spread on a bit of linen and laid over it. The washing and dressing should be repeated twice a day, or more often, if there is much discharge.

When the sides of the wound are torn, the pad should be very carefully washed with boiled water, and when perfectly clean carbolized Vaseline applied on linen.

In bandaging a cut finder use a strip of cotton one inch wide and about twelve inches long. Wind it neatly around the finder and split the end down about three inches – pass one side behind the other and tie it in place. This makes a secure fastening not likely to slip.

After the dressing is removed and the wound almost healed a few narrow strips of adhesive plaster may be laid across it to keep the edges together.

Often a slight cut bleeds profusely, particularly when it is on the head or face. A child comes in from play apparently streaming with blood and when it is washed off with cold water a very trifling injury is revealed.

CUTTING OF A FINGER

If a child has the misfortune to have a finger cut off by a machine, as sometimes happens, the severed member should be picked up, washed in salt water and put in place again, being fastened with strips of adhesive plaster. A bandage should then be wound around it and left undisturbed until the wound heals. If there is a disagreeable odor, or any evidence of inflammation, as redness, heat or swelling, it must be unbound, washed in carbolized water 1-40 and the dressing replaced.

There is good hope that the parts will unite, and at least the experiment ought always to be tried.

Elizabeth Robinson Scovil *The Care of Children*

BLEEDING

If a large blood vessel is cut there will be serious bleeding. If in an arm or leg it can be checked by trying a handkerchief tightly about the limb above the cut, or by putting a thick pad of cotton over the wound and bandaging it very tightly in place. The limb should be raised so the blood will flow backward towards the heart.

Sometimes a piece of ice wrapped in cotton and placed on the bleeding point will control the flow. If the palm is cut the hand can be closed on a piece of ice.

Remember that cold and pressure will almost always stop bleeding and that a good deal of blood can be lost before the danger point is reached.

BLEEDING FROM THE NOSE

If the head is hot and the face congested, bleeding from the nose is sometimes a benefit. When it is profuse the child should sit with the head thrown back, a sponge or wet cloth being held to receive the blood, and something cold put at the back of the neck. Pressing the thumbs on each side of the nose where it joins the lip will control it. If these means fail, gentle syringing with cold salt water is usually effectual.

BLEEDING FROM THE STOMACH

Children sometimes swallow blood from the nose, or gums, and vomit it. It is dark and mixed with food. The symptom is seldom an alarming one. Pieces of ice may be sucked, and the patient made to lie down.

Blood in the motions is usually dark, tarry-looking substance that would scarcely be recognized as such unless one were aware of its peculiar appearance. When it is bright red it often comes from piles.

BLEEDING FROM THE LUNGS

The blood is a bright color and frothy, with bubbles of air through it, and is coughed up.

Raise the head and shoulders with pillows, give bits of ice to suck and, if the pulse is very week, a teaspoonful of brandy in very little water.

Pour a teaspoonful of spirits of turpentine in a pitcher of boiling water and let the steam be inhaled. There is seldom immediate danger.

FOREIGN BODIES IN THE NOSE

Young children are very apt to poke buttons, beaus, beads, and a variety of other small objects into the nose.

Nothing may be said about it at the time and its presence remains undiscovered until inflammation sets in. When there is discharge from one side of the nose only this cause should be suspected.

Gently syringing the nose with warm salt and water, or baking soda and water, will often dislodge the obstruction. The well nostril should be syringed first.

Sometimes a few grains of pepper will cause a sneeze which will bring forth the intruder. If the object is in plain sight efforts may be made to draw it out with a bent hair pin, but poking may injure the delicate membrane and, if not immediately successful, it had better be left to a surgeon.

Foreign Bodies in the Throat

These may be lodged in the windpipe or the food passage.

A quick blow between the shoulder blades, particularly when the child tries to cough, may expel the body. The child may be seized by the feet, held up and shaken.

The finger can be passed into the throat and an effort be made to draw out the obstruction, or, if it is in the food passage, to force it down.

Sometimes the attempt to swallow the white of an egg will loosen the substance so it can be brought up or pushed down. The white should not be beaten.

If immediate relief is not obtained send for the nearest doctor, throw open the window to secure plenty of fresh air and begin artificial respiration.

Swallowing Foreign Bodies

The strong desire that little children must carry everything to their mouths frequently results in foreign substances being swallowed.

A masterly inactivity is the best course to pursue. An object that can pass down the throat can pass through the intestine and probably will do so safely if it is hot interfered with. Even pins may make the journey without doing harm. Emetics and laxatives should not be given. Potato in any form, porridge of oatmeal, rye or wheat, or bread and milk, will form a soft coating around the intruder and conduct it away without injury.

Close watch should be kept for it in the motions. It may not appear for two or three days.

If pain is complained of and there is feverishness or much disturbance, the doctor should be called.

Elizabeth Robinson Scovil *The Care of Children*

SPLINTERS

These should be removed with a sharp needle and usually need no further treatment. If a part remains in the flesh matter will form and a small poultice may be applied until it comes away, when the inflammation will subside, and the spot can be dressed with carbolized Vaseline until it heals.

The mode of dealing with splinters under the nail has already been described.

A fishhook, crochet needle, or any similar instrument with a barbed point, should be pushed through, that it may come out first, not drawn back through the wound.

BRUISE

A flannel wrung out of very hot water laid on a bruise and frequently renewed helps to relieve the soreness. For bruises on the face ice is the best application. Brown paper wet in vinegar is a time-honored remedy. Bathing the part in extract of witch hazel gives relief. After a general contusion, as a fall from a height, a warm bath is soothing.

When the skin is broken the injury is treated as a wound, washed with carbolized water and dressed with carbolized Vaseline.

SPRAINS

These painful accidents are most apt to occur at the wrist, or elbow, knee, or ankle. The ligaments that hold the joints in place are stretched and sometimes torn. It may take longer to recover from a sprain than it does from a bone to unit after it is broken.

Both the hot and cold treatment are recommended. The former is the most soothing for children. Immerse the joint in water as hot as can be borne, keeping up the temperature by adding fresh. Let it soak for an hour or more. Then wrap in warm flannel reinforced by hot-water bags.

As soon as it can be borne, gentle rubbing is useful. Some physicians prescribe perfect rest for the injured part, others active exercise, stopping short of fatigue.

STINGS

The part can be bathed in ammonia or baking soda and water, and a cloth wet in the same bound over it. The sting of a bee can be extracted by pressing the barrel of a small key over it. A handful of moist earth bound on the painful spot often gives ease.

BITES

It is said that, contrary to the usual belief, the bites of the rattlesnake, the moccasin, the copperhead, and one or two other venomous snakes found in this country, are not generally fatal, although the sufferer is profoundly depressed.

Children are more likely to be bitten by dogs, cats, or other pets. The wound should immediately be sucked. It is asserted that there is no danger to the person doing it if the skin of the mouth is unbroken and the saliva is not swallowed.

The wound can be cauterized by heating a buttonhook, or any wire, white-hot and applying it to the surge. The hotter the iron the less the pain. The wound can then be treated as a burn.

If there is much depression, the child should have a little brandy and water.

The animal out to be kept in confinement, provided with food and water and carefully watched. If it does not develop hydrophobia much needless anxiety will be spared. If it does, it is by no means certain that the child will do the same.

Pasteur's method for the prevention of hydrophobia by injecting the virus, properly prepared, has warm advocates. There is an institute in New York where patients can be sent to undergo the treatment, as well as in Paris, where it originated.

BROKEN BONES

The bones of children are so soft that they do not break very easily. When the accident happens, the fracture is often the kind called a green stick fracture. The bone is only partially broken, like a stick of green wood held together by some of the fibers.

The limb must be placed in as natural a position as possible, and the child made comfortable until the doctor comes. It is not necessary that it should be set immediately; delay does no harm. It should be carefully handled not to force the broken ends of the bone through the skin.

When the collarbone is broken the arm is laid across the chest with the hand touching the opposite shoulder and kept in place with a broad bandage or strips of adhesive plaster. It will take about four weeks to unite. With a broken rib a broad bandage is passed around the chest and pinned firmly in place.

DISLOCATIONS

In a dislocation the bone forming the joint is thrown out of the socket. Instead of being unnaturally movable, as when it is broken, the bone is moved with difficulty, there is tenderness and pain. A dislocation should be put back, or reduced, as it is technically called, as soon as possible. If there is much swelling and pain the part can be covered with flannel wrung out of boiling water until the doctor arrives.

BURNS

Burns are of various degrees of severity, from reddening of the part to entire destruction of the tissue.

Almost everyone knows that, as fire cannot burn without air, the most effectual way of putting it out is to wrap the sufferer in a thick woolen rug, blanket, shawl, or piece of carpet. If a child could be dipped under water it would, of course, extinguish the flame; but a little water does no good.

The best remedies to have on hand for burns are baking soda and carbolized Vaseline 1-30.

For slight burns mix the soda to a paste with water and spread it thickly over the part, covering it with linen, or old cotton, secured in place by one or two turns of bandage. This can be kept wet by squeezing tepid water over it.

When there are blisters, they should be carefully pricked, and the fluid absorbed with a piece of soft cotton.

If the shreds of clothing adhere to the burn they should be soaked off with oil, or water, and not pulled off. If the skin is gone, carbolized Vaseline can be spread on linen and bound on the part until the doctor comes.

In severe burns there is a profound shock to the system. The face is pale, the body cold, and the pulse is weak. Put hot-water bags to the feet and over the heart, give brandy in teaspoonful doses, and keep the head low.

A child recovering from an injury of this kind requires careful watching and nourishing food.

In burns caused by acids, water should not be applied to the part; it must be covered with dry baking soda.

If an alkali, as strong ammonia, lye, or quick lime, has done the mischief, use an acid, as vinegar diluted, or lemon juice, to counteract it.

SCALDS

Children are apt to scald themselves by pulling over vessels containing boiling water. The injury should be treated like a burn. When the face is scalded painting it with glycerin sometimes gives relief.

FROST BITES

Frost bites affect the flesh like burns. The frozen part should be rubbed with snow or cold water, that it may thaw gradually, as a too sudden change would destroy its vitality. It should be rubbed persistently but gently until the circulation is restored. Slight cases, as children's usually are, require no further treatment.

FAINTING

Young girls sometimes faint easily. The heart ceases to contract for an instant, cutting off the supply of blood to the brain and unconsciousness follows.

Lay the person down with the head lower than the feet. Either let the head hang over the side of the couch or raise the foot of it on a chair. This usually revives the patient without further treatment.

If not, the dress should be loosened, particularly tight bands about the neck and waist. A few sharp taps may be given over the heart and the face sprinkled with cold water.

If breathing ceases, artificial respiration must be begun.

FITS

These are very often epileptic and occur only in children suffering from epilepsy. The hands are clenched, the sufferer falls unconscious and there may be foam on the lips.

Nothing can be done except to loosen the clothing and guard against the tongue being bitten by putting a spoon, or a tooth-brush handle, or a folded napkin, between the teeth.

All that can be affected by treatment must be done under the physician's direction between the attacks.

CONVULSIONS

Any irritation of the system is very apt to produce convulsions in a young child. Teething and indigestion often bring them on.

The eyes roll, the hands are clenched and there is a general tremor of the whole body.

Remove the clothing quickly and place the child in a hot bath, about 100 degrees Fahrenheit, with a cloth wrung out of cold water on the head. In about two minutes lift him out and roll him in a blanket without wiping him.

Give an enema of warm water and, if the convulsion is soon after a meal, a teaspoonful of wine of ipecac. Putting the finger down the throat will hasten the vomiting.

Convulsions show an irritable condition of the nervous system and are not alarming unless they occur frequently. The child should be kept quiet, and the doctor consulted if they recur.

Elizabeth Robinson Scovil *The Care of Children*

POISONING

Poison Ivy – Children who roam in the woods and fields pick the poison ivy, poison oak, or sumac, which brings out an eruption on the hands and face if it comes in contact with them.

A saturated solution of baking soda, or ammonia and water, will relieve the itching; a cloth soaked in the liquid can be laid over the part and kept wet.

The things to be done, and done quickly when a child has swallowed poison, are:

> To get it out of the stomach,
> To prevent what remains from doing more mischief,
> To counteract the bad effects if possible.

The first thing is to find an emetic. One tablespoon of salt in a glass of tepid water; one dessert-spoonful of mustard, or one teaspoonful of powdered alum kin the same. One teaspoonful of wine of ipecac, followed by lukewarm water. These can be repeated four or five times. Tickling the throat with the finger hastens the action.

Some poisons paralyze the stomach so that it cannot respond to the emetic. If a piece of rubber tubing and a funnel can be procured the tubing can be pushed down the throat, keeping it well at the back, and water poured in through the funnel. Lowering the funnel below the level of the stomach outside, the water runs out. This can be repeated several times, washing it thoroughly.

Neutralizing the poison is accomplished by giving the proper antidote. It is well to administer a dose of castor oil after the danger is over to carry off any remnants of the poison that may have lodged in the intestine.

After a poison that has burned the mouth and throat plenty of milk can be given, flour stirred in water, arrowroot or corn starch gruel.

Opium – Unfortunately, opium is the active ingredient of most of the soothing syrups that some mothers unhesitatingly give their children. Paregoric contains it and laudanum is a strong preparation on it.

A baby under the influence of opium is unnaturally drowsy and sleepy, the breathing is slower than usual, and the pupils of the eyes are very small: nurses sometimes give it to save themselves the trouble, and a mother who has to entrust her children to one should be on the watch for the symptoms.

The baby should be roused and kept awake, if possible. Pour cold water on the head and chest, followed by hot water. An enema of coffee may be given, warm – not hot – and strong. If the breathing is feeble or stops, being artificial respiration. Keep hot bags at the feet and hear and rub vigorously. There are some antidotes a doctor can use which it would not be safe for an unprofessional person to meddle with.

ARSENIC

Children sometimes get at fly poison, which generally contains arsenic.

Give emetic quickly, followed by as much greasy water as can be swallowed. Tablespoonful doses of oil, or oil and lime water, until five or six have been taken. White of egg, flour and water, or any soothing drink. Warmth, hot-water bags, blankets, etc., and rubbing.

OXALIC ACID

In using carbolic acid in any quantity about a wound the urine should be watched and, if dark greenish tinge appears in it, the dressing should be discontinued.

If carbolic acid is swallowed by mistake, a tablespoonful of Epsom salts must be given stirred in water. This is followed by wine of ipecac, or mustard and water, as an emetic. White of egg beaten up in water soothes the irritated membrane.

If there is so much depression that stimulation is needed, apply heat to the feet and over the heart and give brandy in hot water.

PHOSPHORUS

The tops of matches may be bitten off and swallowed. A child is said to have recovered after sucking three hundred. The best emetic is three grains, a very tiny pinch, of sulfate of copper, blue vitriol, dissolved in water; given every five minutes until vomiting occurs. Salt or mustard can be used. Two teaspoonfuls of Epsom salts can be given as a laxative, but no oil nor fat, as that dissolves the phosphorous and makes it easier for the stomach to absorb it.

Children sometimes eat toadstools or poisonous berries, whose nature cannot be determined at the time. An emetic, followed by plenty of milk and later a dose of castor oil, is the best treatment. When the pulse is weak and the face pale, teaspoonful doses of brandy should be given.

DROWNING

Strip off the wet clothes and wrap in a blanket, if possible.

Turn the child on the face over the knee, making pressure over the stomach to expel the water.

Surround the body with hot-water bags, bottles filled with hot water, stove covers wrapped in flannel, or whatever is soonest to be had, taking care not to burn. Keep heat over the heart.

Elizabeth Robinson Scovil *The Care of Children*

Have someone rub the hands, arms, legs and feet unceasingly.

Lay the child on a bed, or table, on the back, see that the tongue is forward in the mouth and begin artificial respiration.

ARTIFICIAL RESPIRATION

Raise the hands above the head; that is, draw them up until the wrists lie on each side of the head, pulling the arms slightly to expand the chest. Bring them down across the chest with a firm pressure to expel the air. Do this slowly sixteen times in the minute, taking two seconds to each movement.

This can be alternated by turning the child first on the face and then on the side at the same rate. The points are:

> To restore breathing;
> To keep up the vital warmth;
> To promote circulation.

The efforts should not be abandoned for at least two hours.

THE EMERGENCY BOX

This should contain the dressings likely to be needed in an emergency and a few simple applications for external use. Liniments and medicines to be given internally never should be kept in the same place.

The following will be found useful:

> An inch-wide roll of rubber adhesive plaster.
> A bunch of absorbent cotton.
> A yard of cheesecloth that has been washed.
> Two rolls of bandage two inches wide and seven yards long,
> made out of an old sheet by sewing the strips together.
> Old cotton.
> Old linen, pieces of tablecloth or napkins.
> Half a yard of thin rubber cloth.
> One dozen safety pins.
> A pair of scissors.
> A small pair of straight dressing forceps.
> Box of carbolized Vaseline 1-30.
> Half a pint of extract of witch hazel.
> Half a pint of spirits of camphor.

Two ounces of spirits of turpentine.
Two ounces of camphorated oil.
A quarter of a pound of boracic acid.
A quarter of a pound of baking soda.
A quarter of a pound of mustard or box of prepared mustard leaves.
Two ounces of good brandy.

Elizabeth Robinson Scovil *The Care of Children*

PHYSICAL CULTURE
CHAPTER XXIII

NECESSITY FOR GYMNASTICS

The ceaseless activity of young children develops their muscles sufficiently without the aid of special exercises.

The baby kicks, creeps, balances himself on his feet and finally walks, meanwhile keeping hands and arms in constant motion, grasping at and playing with every object within reach.

As he grows older, the active games that every healthy child delights in call the muscles into action and promote their growth. It is when they are not used that they become weak and soft.

When a child is cut off from play and forced to sit still for several hours a day, often in a constrained, unnatural attitude, systematic exercise of the muscles becomes a necessity. We call the system of movements devised for this purpose gymnastics.

As we grow in wisdom, no doubt the culture of the body will receive a due share of attention in the schoolroom. The mind cannot be trained and expanded to its fullest capacity unless its companion is able to keep pace with its demands. This it cannot do when some of its parts are allowed to deteriorate from want of use.

In the education of the future competent teachers will be provided to train the body, developing the weak points in the physical frame of each child and strengthening the whole by judicious exercises adapted to its powers.

Until that happy day arrives parents must do as much as possible for the physical development of their children, and what this is must depend a god deal upon the circumstances surrounding them.

Children who live in the country lead an active outdoor life, running, jumping, often rowing, swimming and riding, sometimes engaging in work that calls many muscles into play. There is not such urgent need of gymnastics for these, although it is sometimes found that while the set of muscles most often used is well developed, others, which have not been employed so vigorously, are comparatively undersized.

Children who have no playground but the street, or parks where they are made to keep off the grass, and who do little or no manual labor, have not the opportunity to develop their muscles naturally. For them gymnastics are a very necessary part of the school curriculum and in cities provision should be made for their needs.

What Mothers Can Do

The mother may do much at home if she can devote ten to fifteen minutes every day to the physical training of her children. She must first teach herself what she wishes to teach them, if she has had no special training. Blakie's little book *How to Get Strong* contains much valuable advice. Watson's *Manual of Calisthenics*, although not as recent a work, has one point of advantage, music to which the different exercises can be executed.

Without any special apparatus children can be trained to breathe, stand and walk properly. The muscles of the legs, arms, chest and back can be rounded out until the parts are shapely and firm.

With very inexpensive apparatus, light dumbbells, and a pair of parallel bars, and perhaps a pair of pulley-weights, feats can be accomplished which will give keen pleasure to the children and be of lasting benefit to their rapidly growing bodies.

No one exercise should be prolonged more than two or three minutes and stopped in a shorter time if it fatigues. Practice will enable them to be carried on much longer without this result.

The evening before bedtime is a good opportunity for these exercises if they are not begun to soon after tea.

The clothing just be light and loose. Tight collars and bands, injurious at any time, cannot be tolerated now. Waist, knees, neck and arms must be free. If shoes are worn they must be light and well fitting, not in any way constraining the foot.

Standing

We all know what a frank, fearless look it gives a child to have the head well thrown back and the chin properly poised. A few minutes practice each day standing in a correct attitude helps to render this carriage natural.

The heels should be placed together, the feet turned at right-angles to one another, the knees straight, touching each other, the back straight, shoulders well thrown back, arms hanging easily by the side, palms of the hands turned slightly forward, the neck straight, the chin drawn in, and the eyes a little raised.

Elizabeth Robinson Scovil *The Care of Children*

BREATHING

The importance of breathing through the nose has already been spoken of. Exercise in breathing properly is essential to develop the capacity of the lungs and especially so in children whose chests are weak, or who have an hereditary predisposition to consumption.

Standing in a correct position the mouth should be closed and a long breath taken through the nostrils, exhaling the air slowly by the same channel.

After this has been done several times, the lungs can be filled through the nose and the air expelled through the mouth as forcibly as possible.

Then the air can be inhaled through the nose, the breath held, the arms raised at right angles to the body, the hands placed on the chest and the chest quickly tapped as long as the breath can be held.

Special care must be taken to see that the shoulders are held back, throwing the chest well forward, during these exercises. Also, that the head is erect, and the chin drawn in.

SITTING

An authority on school hygiene has said that "Movement is a child's way of resting; rest is a kind of work to be taught by degrees." Remembering this, we should not expect little children to sit still for long at one time. They should be allowed frequent change of position and to rest by standing and marching about the school room, either to music or without.

A child's chair should support the lower part of the back firmly and comfortably. This is more important than that support should be provided for the shoulders, as much of the time they do not touch the back of the chair.

In school, the desk should be so arranged that stooping is discouraged as much as possible. If the sight is normal, it is easy, after a little practice, to read and write in a correct position with the chest expanded. The head can be bent instead of the shoulders being thrown forward and the back inclined.

The elbows should not rest on the desk as then the shoulders are raised from their proper position.

WALKING

In walking, the body should be held erect, the weight directed rather toward the toes and forward part of the foot. This gives a light springy step, which cannot be acquired if the heel is brought down firmly as the food touches the ground. The knees must be kept back as much as possible and the body below the waistline thrown a little forward.

Running is an excellent exercise for children – races should be encouraged, taking care that they do not take cold afterwards from standing in draughts when they are perspiring and warm.

STRENGTHENING THE MUSCLES

Many exercises have been devised for strengthening the different muscles of the body. By consulting any of the popular books on physical development, the mother will find a description of those best suited to the purpose. There is only room for a few simple ones in a work like this.

Placing the feet together and rising on the toes while the mother counts one, two or plays a bar of music, sinking on the heels and repeating the movements eight or ten times or until fatigued, develops the calf of the leg. While rising on the toes the knees may be bent and straightened again before resting on the heels.

Hopping on one foot is a good exercise; the other may occasionally be bent backward and held in the hand.

Standing firmly on the feet and bending the knees, as if about to kneel, recovering the upright position, and repeating, is a good exercise for the muscles above the knees.

Jumping with a skipping rope assists in developing them, but this should not be overdone.

Dancing also calls them into play and is valuable training for children. It gives them ease and self-confidence and, when well taught, helps to make them graceful.

Standing erect with the knees straight, then bending the body forward trying to touch the floor with the tips of the fingers, helps to strengthen the muscles about the waist. Also, placing the hands on the hips, bending the body first to one side then to the other as far as possible without lifting the feet from the ground.

Holding the head erect with the chin well drawn in, placing the hands behind the neck, extending the arms slowly and bringing them down behind the back with the palms turned out, expands the chest.

Bending the arms until the points of the fingers touch the shoulders and rapidly flexing and extending them; stretching the arms in front with the fists closed, bending them sharply towards the shoulders and letting them drop at the sides with some force, are good arm movements.

Mr. Blakie says that simply opening and shutting the fingers rapidly improves the power of grasping firmly, if faithfully practiced.

In cases of curvature of the spine the surgeon will prescribe gymnastic exercises for remedying the deformity, particularly if the patient is a young child.

STAMMERING

There are few defects more mortifying to the child and more annoying to the friends than stammering, or stuttering. Occasionally it arises from a malformation of the organs of speech. It may be caused by an affection of the mouth, or throat, or some mental deficiency.

Very often it proceeds from nervousness, or a temporary derangement of the health, or is acquired by imitating another child thus afflicted. It is more catching than measles.

It does not usually manifest itself in children under four years old.

Whispering and singing do not present the same difficulties as speaking, the child rarely stammering then.

The utmost patience, gentleness ad perseverance are necessary in training children with this defect. Very much can be accomplished by persistent painstaking; the effort must be continuous and not abandoned because there is little improvement for a long time.

It is very important to enforce correct habits of breathing through the nose. The lungs should be filled before beginning to speak.

Speaking slowly must be insisted upon and when there is a stammer, the child should stop and slowly and quietly repeat the difficult word, or letter. The sounds that lie most often trips upon should be practiced again and again, filling the lungs before each attempt and repeating then deliberately until for once he can say them smoothly. The knowledge that he can do so gives him confidence in future trials.

Standing erect and inhaling a long breath he can give different vowel sounds, as ah, ee, ih, oh, ooh, holding each as long as possible. Then the vowels and consonants combined, in such words as ail, ebb, ice, old, up, etc.

When the stammer comes, always stop the speaker and insist on his taking time to recover himself, fill his lungs and try again, instead of vainly trying to enunciate the word without stopping to breathe.

Attention should be paid to the general health and the nervous system. Sleep and diet are factors in the treatment not to be neglected.

THE CARE OF GIRLS
CHAPTER XXIV

THE MENSTRUAL PERIOD

Until a girl is ten years old her life may be much the same as her brothers'. She should be encouraged to spend a good deal of time out of doors, to run, play active games, and take plenty of exercise. This contributes to her physical development and enables her to lay up a store of strength for the years to come.

The menstrual period comes much earlier to some girls than to others. It is usually preceded by mental and bodily disturbances more or less well defined. In a strong, healthy girl these may be very slight. With more delicate ones there are nervous symptoms, often irritability and unreasonableness without apparent cause, and vague sensations of discomfort, hardly defined enough to be called pain, and yet disturbing and distressing.

Infinite patience and tenderness is needed in dealing with these cases. The child does not mean to be naughty, and her feelings are as much a problem to herself as they are to her mother, who often does not recognize a physical cause for the ill humor she finds it hard to condone.

It is inexcusable that a girl should be allowed to approach this period without having its meaning explained to her. Well instructed mothers do not leave their children to find out the great facts of life from ignorant companions, who strip them of their sacredness and make what God has ordained common and unclean.

If fathers and mothers were frank with their boys and girls, telling them modestly and truthfully the things that they ought to know and warning them against dangers into which they may fall from ignorance, much sin, anguish of mind and suffering of body would be saved.

Why should not the questions that all children ask sooner or later, be candidly answered? They are conscious of no impropriety in asking them and there is none in answering them with the same fidelity to truth that we show in explaining any fact to them as far as they can understand it.

Nothing so rapidly and fatally destroys a child's confidence in his parents as to find that they have deceived him, and girls are fully sensitive on this point as boys.

Elizabeth Robinson Scovil *The Care of Children*

The unthinking jest, or subterfuge, that stopped or satisfied the inquirer for the moment, is looked back upon, when fuller knowledge comes, with a resentment that parents would find it hard to understand unless they can remember vividly the experiences of their own childhood.

REST

This is one of the most important factors in the treatment of a girl, not only during the establishment of the menstrual function, but during all the years of school life until she is fully developed.

For the first year the child should be kept quiet during these days, made to lie down for a few hours and not allowed to indulge in any violent exercise.

Tennis, riding on horse-back, rowing, swimming, must always be given up for the time being. Long walks should not be taken, hard study prohibited, and the girl trained to take care of herself at this time. Dancing is injurious; although an occasional indulgence in this pastime might not do harm, it should not be a habitual amusement under these circumstances.

COLD

Cold is an enemy especially to be dreaded and the feet are an extremely vulnerable point. With most girls it is a serious matter to get the feet wet. Should it happen, they must be well rubbed with spirits of camphor or alcohol, dried and kept in warm stockings.

An extra wrap should be worn, and every precaution taken against a chill, or any exposure to draughts. If obliged to go out in damp weather, a cloak should be put on and the dress changed on coming in if it is not perfectly dry.

BATHING

A plunge bath must never be taken while the flow continues. The feet should not be dipped into a basin of water, but washed with a cloth and thoroughly rubbed until the blood circulates briskly through them. In taking a sponge bath the water should be warm and a part of the body washed and dried before proceeding farther, the parts that are not actually being washed kept covered.

The room must be comfortably warm.

CLOTHING

As already stated, a girl's clothing must be loose, comfortable, and not too heavy.

Grace, beauty and health all demand the absence of tight bands, or any constriction about the waist.

Sanitary towels can now be purchased to take the place of napkins. These are used once and then destroyed. They cost about sixty cents a dozen and can be made more cheaply of cotton waste and cheese cloth. The latter must be washed to render it soft enough to use. An elastic girdle is the most comfortable, it can be about an inch wide, fastened with small button and buttonhole.

In cold weather it is an advantage to a delicate girl to wear a flannel binder. A straight strip rolls up unless kept in place by straps. But a pattern of a well-fitting one can be obtained from any establishment that deals in paper patterns.

Coincident Symptoms

The breasts, enlarging at this time, sometimes become tender and a little painful. The dress should not be allowed to press upon them. The tenderness can be relieved by soaking a handkerchief in spirits of camphor and laying it across them.

Backache should not manifest itself in a healthy girl. If it does, unless very severe, it does not require treatment. A mustard paste, one part mustard to two of flour, left on until the skin is reddened, helps to relieve it.

Sometimes severe abdominal pain is felt for a time during the early stage. A hot-water bag is comforting. If this does not relieve, poultices or hot fomentations may be tried. A teaspoonful of tincture of ginger in hot water is beneficial. Alcohol and opium should never be given to a girl without a physician's prescription. If the pain is serious enough to seem to require these remedies a doctor ought to be consulted.

Delayed Menstruation

After the function is established, the periods ought to recur about once in four weeks. With some perfectly healthy persons the interval is shorter. When the flow does not come at the expected time, a day or two of grace should be allowed, as cold, over-exertion, mental anxiety, or any over-strain, may delay its appearance. The feet can be soaked in hot water and a tumbler of hot lemonade taken at bedtime. A sitz bath, in which the girls sits in a tub of water with the feet outside and covered with a blanket, is efficacious.

If the flow is long delayed, there may be bleeding from the nose, spitting of blood, or, sometimes, vomiting it from the stomach. This is not specially alarming, being nature's compensation, or vicarious menstruation, as it is called.

During the first year or two, the periods may intermit for two or three months at a time without serious consequences.

There is often constipation, which should be relieved by licorice powder, or any mild laxative.

Elizabeth Robinson Scovil *The Care of Children*

If a girl does not menstruate by the time she is fifteen a physician should be consulted.

HYSTERIA

Girls of a nervous temperament are apt to have a variety of symptoms at this time which are included under this general term. There may be fits of excessive laughter, or crying, a general want of self-control, shown in acts of wanton mischief, fits of unprovoked ill-temper and apparent attacks of fainting or convulsions. These can be distinguished from true faintness, or fits, by two symptoms. The girl never hurts herself, as by biting her tongue, or striking her head in falling, and the eyes are sensitive, which is not the case when a person is unconscious. If an attempt is made to open the lids she resists, trying to keep them shut, and flinches if the eyeball is touched with the finger.

This attempted deceit is a part of her mental and physical condition, for which she is not fully responsible. Medical treatment is necessary, tonics, nourishing food, baths, gentle exercise, sleep, and all hygienic measures, to restore tone to the system.

At the same time, her moral nature should be appealed to, and a desire to struggle against her weakness be awakened in her. Girls have a great longing for sympathy, and while this should be lovingly given, it must be directed to the causes that have brought about this condition of weakness, and not to the symptoms of it. She must be made to understand that self-control is a virtue, and that a girl who willfully gives way to foolish manifestations loses the respect of right-thinking persons.

During the attack, a judicious letting-alone is the most efficacious treatment. Often the mention of a disagreeable remedy, as asafetida, or a douche of cold water, will cut it short. Rest in a darkened room should be enforced afterwards.

Contrary to the general belief, boys sometimes suffer from an hysterical condition, as well as girls, and even men have been known to be afflicted with it.

SCHOOL WORK

Girls seldom break down from over-study alone. If properly treated, the body is usually capable of meeting the demands upon it. When it is underfed, stinted in sleep and expected to respond to calls in too many different directions at once, it rebels.

Then we have pale faces, headache, backache, and nervous prostration, with all its attendant ills.

The trouble lies, not in over-study, but in overstrain. Mothers must remember that girls cannot go to school and meet the claims of society at the same time.

Late hours are absolutely incompatible with keeping the young, growing body in good condition.

A schoolgirl should not be allowed to go to parties in the evening, except possibly occasionally on Friday night.

If she is permitted to go to the theatre, matinees should be chosen. A concert in the evening at rare intervals may be permissible.

If a girl is restrained in these outside pleasures and made to live her life more slowly she is a gainer in the end. She gains in freshness what she loses in present gratification. She has not exhausted all forms of entertainment by the time she is eighteen, and when she emancipated from the school room she brings to social functions a capacity for enjoyment that is in proportion to their novelty.

If a girl wishes to go to college she wants to take their unimpaired health, steady nerves, and the power of close application. This she cannot do unless her physical well-being has been carefully attended to during the formative period of earlier youth.

NEEDLE WORK

A girl who cannot sew neatly and quickly misses an important accomplishment. The taste for it must be cultivated and the mother must not begin by making it unattractive to the little learner.

The second occupation in kindergarten work is a kind of coarse embroidery with colored worsted on cardboard pricked in different patterns to permit the passage of the needle.

This does for a beginning and may be followed by working with worsted on canvas. When the child has learned to handle the needle easily a smaller one can be substituted and the first lessons in over-handing given.

The seams should be short, the fabric pretty and the work made as fascinating as possible.

Excellent paper patterns for dolls' clothes can be procured from the dealers in paper patterns. With these, cutting out the tiny garments can be made an interesting pastime. The proper way of placing the pattern on the material, the care necessary to ensure perfect accuracy, and many other useful lessons, can be taught by their means.

As the girl grows older, she should learn to cut and fit her own dresses. There are several admirable systems of measurement which make the work easier than it used to be it was more empirical.

Elizabeth Robinson Scovil *The Care of Children*

If she has any taste for the millinery, it should be cultivated, and lessons taken in the art. In many large cities there are classes where instruction is given, and even in smaller places, there is usually someone who is able and willing to impart the necessary knowledge for a consideration.

A girl who can cut and make her own clothes, trim her own hats, and those of other people, if necessary, is independent. If reverses come, she is prepared to meet them.

Any girl can earn her own living who can do *well* what everyone wants to have done.

If is cruel to bring a girl up without giving her perfect command of some useful art which she can turn to account in time of need.

Every mother should choose one for her daughter and see that she is perfected in it, whatever it may be. If she never requires using it to gain her daily bread, it will still be a desirable accomplishment, and, in the changes that life brings, it may be a sheet anchor that saves her from destruction.

Housework

There is no better exercise for young girls than a moderate amount of housework. It develops the muscles, improves the circulation, and so the complexion; and, if it roughens the hands, a little Vaseline, or glycerin and rose water, with a pair of gloves worn at night, counteracts the ill effect.

A knowledge of cooking is invaluable to a girl. How to purchase and prepare food so it may yield the largest amount of nutriment for the smallest expenditure of money, should be a part of her training.

There are many good books on cookery which can be used to supplement the personal teaching.

A mother should be ashamed to send her daughter to be the housemother in any man's home, if she is deficient in the housewifely arts in which it was her duty to instruct her.

Homemaking is the primary business of a woman's life, and she ought to understand the arts that lie at its foundation. She will find ample opportunity to practice them, if it is only to make a home for herself in one room.

Should her sphere be a wider one, she will have the satisfaction of filling it with ease and can command efficient service, because she knows what she requires and can supplement deficiencies by proper instruction.

Most people like to do what they can do well, and girls are no exception to the general rule. The mother must be patient with failures and not give to scanty a measure of praise when it is deserved. The efforts to render service that is sometimes more hindrance than help must be accepted and encouraged. It is much easier to do things oneself than to teach others to do them, but training is the mother's mission, and she must fulfil it faithfully in small things as well as great.

Saturday morning is a good time to devote to the special lessons in housekeeping. If some triumph of cookery can appear at the festival dinner on Sunday, the family approval will be a reward the young maker will remember all her life.

PREPARING GIRLS FOR BOARDING SCHOOL

The question of whether or not to send a girl to boarding school is a vexed one. It seems a pity that she should ever have to be sent away from her parents. They are her natural guardians, and no one can adequately fill their places.

When a girl's home is in the country, where she cannot have suitable educational advantages without leaving it, sending her away seems to be a necessity, if it is impossible to employ a governess. Sometimes the stimulus of companionship in study is necessary.

When circumstances arise to render it desirable, the school should not be chosen because it is large, or fashionable, or cheap, but an earnest endeavor should be made to find one where the personal influence of the principal may be counted upon as an element of good in the formation of the child's character.

Many noble women have been at the head of these institutions whose uprightness and singleness of purpose, purity of mind and fidelity to duty, have left an impression upon their pupils' lives whose value it would be hard to over-estimate.

Much depends upon the spirit in which the girl goes to meet her new opportunity. The mother may give wise and loving counsel that will greatly help her in the untried life, so different from the seclusion of home.

She should be especially cautioned in regard to her health and charged to go to those in authority if she is out of order, not to let constipation persist when a laxative would give relief, and to take the same care of herself that she has been accustomed to do at home. Some of the larger schools have a trained nurse in charge of the infirmary, to whom the girls may go at any time for advice and treatment for slight ailments.

She will gain much more from the training if she goes in an obedient spirit, realizing that rules are not made at the caprice of the teachers but for the benefit of the girls, and that to break them for fun not only does not bring much enjoyment in the end, but is a distinct injury to herself.

Elizabeth Robinson Scovil *The Care of Children*

In choosing a school one should be selected where the pupils are well fed. Growing girls, especially when their brains are being taxed, need a varied and abundant diet. This point being satisfactorily settled, the mother should refrain from sending boxes of eatables. A little candy may be allowed now and then – if it is home-made so much better – but a quantity of promiscuous sweets only does harm. Many of the wisest principals will not permit them to be received.

The mother should insist that the home letters are to be free from surveillance and the girl should be encouraged to write freely. While being careful not to interfere between the pupil and the constituted authority, many misunderstandings may be smoothed out by a little advice from the calmer judgment of the elder, and many questions settled by helping the child to bring them to the touchstone of right or wrong.

The clothing that is necessary varies with the season of the year and the length of the term.

Four changes of underclothing are sufficient, as more can be supplied from the additional stock at home should they be needed. It is well to send six pairs of stockings. A pair of walking boots, two pairs of house shoes, slippers and rubbers should be provided.

A bottle of shoe dressing containing glycerin should be carried in the traveling bag. The consequences of a breakage are too disastrous to trust it in the trunk.

Extra shoelaces must not be forgotten.

Two school dresses of some pretty, soft woolen material, a plain serge traveling dress, another rather more elaborate for Sunday, and a fine, light cashmere, challis, or India silk for evening wear or festival occasions, is an ample supply of dresses. A warm wrapper of Jersey or eiderdown flannel, a pretty dressing jacket of outing or opera flannel, and a pair of bedroom slippers should be included in the outfit.

If tennis is played, a tennis suit will be required, and tennis shoes. Possibly a suit for gymnastic exercises as well.

It is nice to have two or three cambric shirt waists for the first warm days in early summer. A girl loves fresh, dainty things and, while she should not be encumbered with a number of dresses for unnecessary display, she should have enough to keep her trim and comfortable.

A thick jacket, or warm ulster, is necessary for the daily outing, and a pretty hat, felt in winter, and straw in summer, not to elaborately trimmed. A second hat should be provided for state occasions.

A girl should not be stinted in gloves. Three or four pairs are required, as she is obliged to wear them in the daily constitutional walk, and they soon grow shabby. A muff is a comfortable addition in winter.

A desk, well-furnished with paper, envelopes, pens and postage stamps, the latter in a little case with leaves of waxed paper, should be one of the parting gifts, if it is not already counted amongst the valued possessions. A lock and key are indispensable.

A workbag, with all the accessories for sewing ready at hand, must not be omitted. Besides the sewing implements there should be extra buttons of every kind used in the wardrobe, shoe and glove buttons, sewing cotton, mending silk, strong linen thread for sewing on boot buttons, beside the ordinary black and white spools. Tape and a bodkin are useful, and a box of patent button-fasteners enables a missing boot button to be replaced quickly. A shoe-bag for the closet door, two clothes-bags and a hanging-case for umbrella and sun-umbrella should be added.

A napkin ring is always taken, and in some schools the pupils are required to bring two silver forks, a teaspoon, a dessertspoon and tablespoon.

Too many belongings are burdensome, but the girl should have a standing frame for the home photographs, a toilet cushion, and a few pretty things to adorn her room.

All her clothing should be plainly marked, the underclothing with her full name. The umbrella may have a tag with the name sewn to one of the ribs inside, if she is not fortunate enough to have a silver plate engraved with her initials.

A good-sized trunk must be provided to hold the equipment. It is well if the lock has two keys, one to be kept at home and sent in case of emergency.

A traveling bag is needed and a strap to hold umbrella and parasol together is convenient.

A watch is a comfort to a girl at school who is old enough to take care of it. Very pretty silver ones, either chatelaine or plain, can be obtained at such a moderate cost that they can usually be afforded with comparative ease.

Handsome jewelry should be left behind in safe keeping. It is always unsuitable for young girls, and never more so than at school. Two, or three, pretty pins are all that is needed.

The amount of picket money permitted is usually regulated by the principal of the institution, and her judgment in the matter should not be questioned. If a girl has had an allowance and been taught to manage it judiciously, the responsibility of spending money will not be a new thing to her. There is no reason why girls should not be taught to keep accounts and conduct their small affairs systematically, in preparation for the duties of later years.

Elizabeth Robinson Scovil *The Care of Children*

A Daughter's Privileges

The instinct of every true mother is to spend herself for the benefit of her children. So strong is the impulse that she must be careful lest it lead her into sacrificing herself in such a way as to injure rather than to serve them.

When a mother foregoes her own claim to consideration, puts herself in the background, abdicates her rightful place as the chief authority in her household and allows her daughter to usurp her privileges, she does the girl a cruel wrong.

Deference belongs to the mother by rights of her position, and she must exact it from her children. They may have had greater advantages than she has had, but, while this may increase her pride in them, it must not alter the natural relation.

A mother must above all things keep the respect of her children, and this she cannot do she always takes the lower place and allows them to rule her household.

It is a daughter's privilege especially to be her mother's right hand, serving and sparing her in every way that love can devise. If this service is always exacted as a tribute of love it will never be felt a burden. Instead of a mother invariably taking upon herself the hard tasks or disagreeable duties, it will be the daughter's pleasure to assume some of them and let the weight rest on the strong young shoulders, where a part a least of it belongs.

Children are always proud to be able to help their mother. The training should be begun early, the childish efforts met with warm approval and loving appreciation, and the habits so formed will not be discontinued in later years.

It is a daughter's privilege to be able to invite her friends to her home, but the mother is the hostess in her own house. It is she who must receive and welcome the guests and make it plain that she regards them as hers as well as her daughter's friends.

A house where visitors come and go unseen and unwelcomed by the mistress of it is not one where the careful mother would desire her children to be intimate.

It is a daughter's especial privilege to be the companion and caretaker of her father. The tie between them is very strong and she should strive in every way in her power to repay him for all he has done for her. She brings a brightness into his life, often clouded by business cares and worries, of which she has no conception. She should cultivate all the little ways of pleasing him that she has found to be successful. She should submit cheerfully even to restriction for which she cannot understand the necessity, because she does not know the reasons that lie behind them.

Perhaps the mother never is as proud of the daughter she has watched and trained with such tender, careful guidance as when she sees her great comfort to her father as she is to herself.

THE CARE OF BOYS
CHAPTER XXV

YOUTH

The change from boyhood to youth is much slower in boys than the corresponding period in girls. The friends do not always remember that the awkwardness and bashfulness, the tendency to uncomfortable blushing, the irritability and moodiness that often accompany it, are nervous manifestations to be dealt with considerately.

The father can do much to guide his boy at this time, and he should not neglect his duty towards him.

Good food, active outdoor games, a cheerful home atmosphere, and pleasant associates, help a boy through this transition period as he passes on to the responsibilities of manhood.

PREPARING BOYS FOR BOARDING SCHOOL

This is not a serious matter as preparing girls for a similar goal. Boys do not require as many adjuncts to make them comfortable as their sisters do, and, yet, some thought must be expended upon the outfit.

The under clothing should be in good condition, if not perfectly new, as the mending is usually provided for at the school, and it is not fair to impose an unnecessary burden by sending it half worn and ready to break into holes.

A plentiful supply of socks should be provided, at least eight pairs, and renewed during the term, as long tramps and violent physical exercise are very hard on foot gear.

Two strong suits of clothes, with a couple of extra pairs of trousers and a finer suit for Sunday, will be needed. A pea-jacket, or reefer, is desirable for wet weather. An overcoat is necessary, and a muffler and mittens in cold weather.

Stout shoes and rubber boots must be provided to protect the feet, and a lighter pair for the house.

A boy should be well furnished with the smaller accessories of the toilet, neckties, an extra pair of suspenders, and a supply of collars, studs and shirt buttons.

A mending bag will not be out of place for him, if he has learned to use its contents.

Elizabeth Robinson Scovil *The Care of Children*

A box containing brushes and blacking for his boots will be appreciated after he has struggled with those that are common property.

He will probably need a gymnasium suit and shoes.

In some schools the boys are required to furnish their cubicles, or small divisions of the large dormitory, one of which is assigned to each boy. In this case, strong, plain furniture should be chosen, and can usually be obtained from a dealer near the school who makes a business of providing it.

Unless there is a lavish supply of blankets, a small down comforter is a welcome addition to the bedcovering in winter.

It is very mortifying to a boy not to be able to have the things which his companions have and consider necessaries. While extravagance should be discouraged, a boy's requests should be listened to with attention, carefully considered, and granted if there is no good reason against it.

Skates, tennis rackets, baseball bat, sleds, the many implements that are needed for games and diversions of various kinds, mean little to the elders who have left them far behind. Their possession makes all the difference between affluence and poverty to a boy whose little world has agreed to consider them indispensable.

If it is impossible to afford them, the reason should be frankly explained to the boy. It will not make it easier for him to do without them, but it will remove any trace of bitterness at being denied them.

The Children's Companions

There are few things in the education of her children that cause the thoughtful mother more anxiety than the influence exerted over them by the companions amongst whom they are thrown.

A bad boy, or girl, in a few hours, or days, can do more harm than can be remedied in months, or years.

There is no safeguard except in constant watchfulness and in keeping unbroken the confidence of the children.

The mother whose children turn to her naturally in all their troubles and pleasures, who bring to her their perplexities to be resolved and their triumphs to be sympathized with and rejoiced over, need not so much fear the enemy who would poison their minds with evil.

The thought of her trust in them, the certainty that she will listen to whatever they have to say with respectful attention and will give satisfactory answers to their inquiries, treating them as children love to be treated, like reasonable beings, is the strongest protection that she can throw around them.

We cannot shield children from temptations, not protect them absolutely from contact with evil. We can only prepare them as far as lies in our power to resist and overcome.

The mother should make friends of the companions of her children, showing an interest in their pleasures and pursuits and trying to obtain their confidence. In this way she will be able to judge of their temper and disposition, and if she sees that their intercourse is likely to do harm, she can discourage it.

Children respond very readily to a real interest in their affairs. They can see as quickly as their elders when anyone is willing to take trouble to please them and it is not difficult to win their hearts. Youth is the time to make friends; they often are the possession of a lifetime. The childish friendship, that has grown and ripened with years, has a peculiar flavor that no later one can have. The mother should see that her child has an opportunity to cultivate friends, and, as circumstances many convert them into lifelong ones, as far as possible the companions from whom they must be selected should be wisely chosen.

Children should be encouraged to ask their friends to share the games, or listen to the reading, or music, that makes the home evening pleasant.

Boys particularly should be made to feel that home is as free and happy as any place in the world; that friends are always welcome, unless there is some temporary cause that makes it inconvenient to have them at a special time. Their tastes should be consulted and their wishes deferred to within reasonable bounds. While never usurping the first place, which belongs of right to the parents, they are important members of the family, and should be treated as such.

Reading

A taste for reading gives great pleasure through life. Persons who have the happy faculty of losing themselves in a book, forgetting worries and troubles for the time being, are to be envied.

As a resource in old age, it is without equal. It is possessed by children in a very varying degree and, like other tastes, can be cultivated. Some children learn to read almost imperceptibly, seeming to acquire that art without much definite instruction. To others, the accomplishment means a long struggle and many tears.

If a child can be interested in a story, he may be allured by the prospect of being able to read it himself. Children's books are so fascinating nowadays that it seems an easy task to awaken an interest in them.

As children grown beyond the baby books, they should not be allowed to read stories exclusively. There are many elementary books in the different branches of science that are well within the comprehension of children from eight years old.

Elizabeth Robinson Scovil *The Care of Children*

If their curiosity is aroused, they will be anxious to learn something about the birds, animals, insects and plants that surround them and to know something of the construction of their own wonderful bodies.

Mr. George E. Hardy, of New York, prepared a graded and annotated list, called *Five Hundred Books for the Young*, which has been published in book form and gives much valuable information as to the best books for children.

To be read to is usually an unfailing source of delight. The little ones will listen to the same story again and again, seeming to find fresh pleasure in every repetition. If the mother can read to the flock for half an hour every evening it is surprising what a number of books can be enjoyed in the course of a year.

As soon as children have mastered the difficulty of comprehending printed words they should be encouraged to read aloud. It is possible to teach a little child, who has not acquired bad habits of artificial intonation, to read as simply and naturally as he speaks.

Reading aloud agreeably is a delightful accomplishment and ought to be as spontaneous as speaking, no more and no less difficult; yet how few possess it. The moment the average child attempts to interpret the pages of a book, or the columns of a newspaper, the voice becomes strained and harsh, the utterance hurried or indistinct, and the performance, far from giving pleasure to the listener, is usually a source of annoyance and discomfort.

The books that a child reads have much to do with the formation of his ideals, although he would not dream of using so ambitious a word himself. The standard of his favorite hero affects his own in no small measure. To an imaginative girl her companions in books area as real as those she meets in her daily life, and she unconsciously imitates their virtues or defects and is influenced by their actions.

No mother should permit her children to read books of which she knows nothing. If she has not time to peruse them herself, she must choose them under the guidance of a competent authority, a friend in whom she has confidence, or a book review on which she can rely.

Some authors she knows can be depended upon, not only in the important matters of purity and right views of life, but for a grace of style, a correctness of diction, and a sunniness of outlook that make their books as charming as they are improving.

Let the children learn to cultivate the dear book friends, who never grow old nor change, and who, when they turn to them in after years, will still have the power to recall somethings of the sweetness of the childish days when they were first known and loved.

Home Training

The wise mother will let her boys share in some of the training that she gives her girls. It does not hurt a boy to know how to make his own bed, darn his own stockings, or even cook his own dinner. The time may come when he will be thankful that he is able to do so, and, in any case, a knowledge of the difficulties to be overcome will make him more lenient towards the failures of others.

It is not easy for a mother to share in the pursuits of her boys as it is in those of her girls, so she should make the most of those that they can have in common.

Collections are invaluable as a means of exciting a boy's interest. It does not much matter what the material is, so long as it serves for a starting-point and opens up fresh avenues of thought.

Postage stamps are the most common at present. They exercise the powers of observation, as it often requires close scrutiny to distinguish between the different issues. They may lead to a greater interest in geography and history and are not to be despised as educators.

Collections of stones, mosses, flowers, the different kinds of wood, etc., open the way to a knowledge of many interesting branches of natural history.

Observing and recording the habits of birds and animals, distinguishing the different species of butterflies and other insects, in short, a loving interest in the works and ways of nature, is a distinct source of pleasure and advantage, not only in youth, but through the whole of life.

A happy childhood is the right of every child. Restrictions there must be to protect children from harm and to help them to do right. These should not be made needlessly galling, nor, on the other hand, must freedom degenerate into license.

Love and confidence should be the ruling spirit of the family life. The wise mother holds in her keeping the hearts of her household and guides them so gently they scarcely know they are being ruled.

Many faults will be outgrown almost imperceptibly; many defects will seem to correct themselves under her gentle touch. If she exacts truthfulness and obedience to the laws of right, not always to her own will, she may leave many minor matters to take care of themselves.

If she keeps her own standard high, her ideals will impress themselves upon her children and they will never be satisfied with lower ones.

Elizabeth Robinson Scovil *The Care of Children*

INDEX

A

Abdomen 58, 118-119, 121, 127-128, 136, 139-140, 158, 164
Abdominal pain 186
Accidents 85, 168, 171
Acids 26, 173
Ailments 7, 15, 51, 97, 117, 119, 190
Air 12, 25, 35, 47, 62, 76-79, 89, 92, 98, 101-102, 123-124, 127, 132, 137, 143-147, 156, 160-161, 165-166, 169-170, 173, 177, 181
Albumen 42-43
Alcohol 24, 27, 46, 105, 115, 159, 167, 185-186
Alkaline 29
Alum 24, 94, 124, 133, 155, 175
Ankles 64, 114, 162
Appetite 27, 33, 54, 98, 144, 152, 157-158
Aprons 11, 72

Arms 58, 72, 82, 86, 88, 92, 114, 126, 137, 141, 145-146, 149, 177, 179-182
Arrowroot 10, 36, 52, 175
Arsenic 20, 176
Artificial light 13, 96, 98
Asthma 19, 161-162
Astigmatism 96-97
Atomizer 155

B

Babyhood 7, 11, 68, 76
Bacon 9, 43, 48, 54, 56
Baked apple 41, 48, 133
Bananas 44
Bandages 136
Bands 10, 57-58, 62, 66, 70, 76, 85, 119, 174, 180, 185
Bangs 14, 106
Barley 8, 26, 30-31, 36-37, 52-54, 159

C

Flaxseed poultice 130
Flour ball 9, 36, 52
Fomentations 17, 125,
    147, 155, 162, 186
Fontanelle 164
Freckles 17, 142
Fresh milk 33
Frost bites 20, 173
Fruit 9, 41-42, 44-45, 48-51, 159
Fumigation 17, 149, 155

G

Garments 11, 57-58, 60,
    72-73, 81-82, 188
Gavage 17, 146
Gelatine 9, 40
Germs 32, 84, 159, 166
Girls 11, 20-21, 68-73,
    79, 106, 137, 163, 174,
    184-192, 194, 198
Glands 17, 105, 123, 141-
    142, 152, 157, 166
Glasses 96-98, 132
Graham bread 51
Gravies 49
Grinding the teeth 13, 94
Growing pains 16, 130
Gruel 9, 26, 31, 36-38,
    52-54, 144, 175
Gum boils 15, 124
Gymnastics 20, 179-180

H

Hair 14, 60, 76-77, 105-109, 127,
    130, 142, 148, 150-151, 170
Hammocks 11, 76
Hampers 12, 80
Hands 16, 59, 63, 85, 91, 95, 110,
    112, 114, 118, 128, 131, 147-
    148, 150, 155, 159-160, 163,
    174-175, 177, 179-182, 189
Hang nails 111
Hare lip 16, 137
Harsh hair 14, 107
Headache 16, 27, 97, 106, 131-
    132, 154, 158, 162, 187
Heat rash 54, 126
Heel 15, 67, 70, 116, 181
Hemorrhoids 140
Hernia 139-140
Hiccough 15, 121
Hip disease 16, 136
Hives 54, 126
Hoarseness 15, 122, 156, 161
Hold 33, 35, 43, 48, 70, 75, 80, 84-
    85, 103, 114, 121, 124, 171, 192
Home training 21, 198
Hominy 38, 54, 56, 165
Hopping 182
Hot-water bag 118, 129-
    130, 165, 167, 186
Housework 20, 189
Hysteria 20, 187

Bibliographies of the Editors

Jonathan Savage was born in Portland, Maine, U.S.A. He was adopted at birth, joining his new parents who were living in Sao Paulo, Brazil. Eventually, his family also lived in Peru, Ecuador, Colombia, and Venezuela. Jonathan returned to the United States to attend Wheaton College in Wheaton, Illinois, and then the University of Illinois College of Law in Chicago, Illinois.

After graduation from law school, Jonathan worked as an international lawyer at Baker McKenzie in Chicago. There, he represented Fortune 400 companies doing business in Central and South America, and Spain. Next, Jonathan dove into investment banking at A.G. Edwards & Sons, Inc. and there rose to the position of Member of the Board of Directors and Head of the public finance investment banking division. Finally, Jonathan returned to the legal profession as a United States securities and municipal-bond finance attorney and continues to practice law.

༺༻

At Iowa State University's College of Design **Mikesch Muecke**, a German-born designer and creator, teaches interdisciplinary studios in preservation and cultural heritage, architecture studios on topics intersecting with his own research agenda (currently film and architecture), history/theory/practice seminars, and digital media courses in the Architecture Department.

He holds a Ph.D. in Architectural History and Theory (1999) and a post-professional Master of Science in Architecture (1995), both from Princeton

University, as well as a professional Master of Architecture (1991) and Bachelor of Design with a Major in Architecture (1989) from the University of Florida. He is principal of polytekton, a design/build practice that's part of a larger network of companies engaged with the built environment in its physical, historical, cultural, theoretical, and temporal representations.

Mikesch is an award-winning founder and owner of Culicidae Press/Culicidae Architectural Press, a peer-reviewed publishing house specializing in biographies and design books, as well as four other imprints (Handcar Press, Hog Press, Zanzara Press, and Musca Press) for which he edits, designs, and publishes books in electronic, paperback, and hardcover versions that are available worldwide.

≪❧≫

Judy Berthiaume practiced as a licensed nurse for over forty years. Twenty of those years were spent working specifically with children as a pediatric nurse. In her practice, Judy focused on both the physical and emotional well being of her 'children'. And, as the children grew and healed, she loved them — and they loved her back.

www.ingramcontent.com/pod-product-compliance
Lightning Source LLC
Chambersburg PA
CBHW052111020426
42335CB00021B/2712